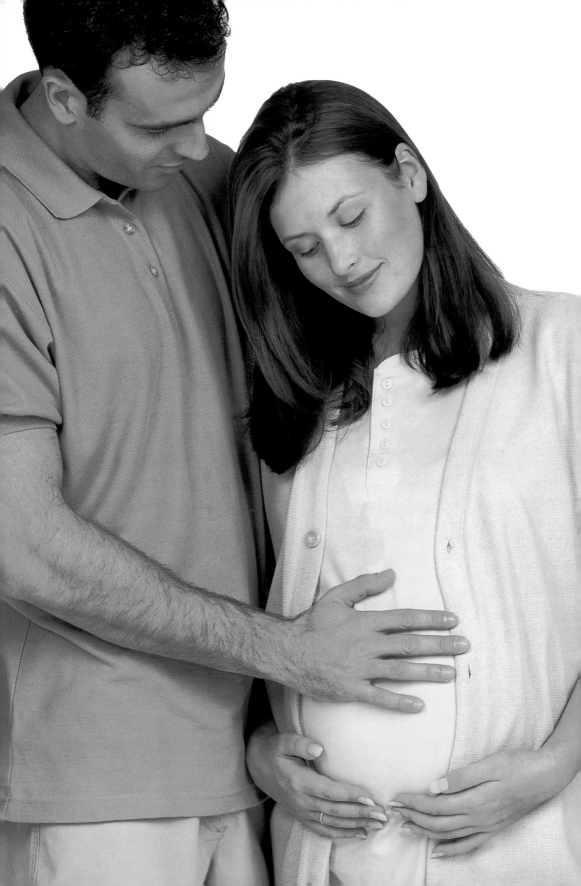

The Pregnancy QUESTION &ANSWER *Book*

Dr Christoph Lees BSc MRCOG

Dr Karina Reynolds FRCSEd MRCOG

Grainne McCartan RGN RM BSc

DORLING KINDERSLEY

LONDON • NEW YORK • SYDNEY • MOSCOW
www.dk.com

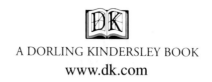

A DORLING KINDERSLEY BOOK
www.dk.com

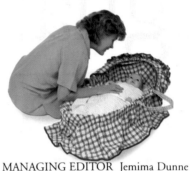

MANAGING EDITOR Jemima Dunne

PROJECT EDITOR Jacqueline Jackson

EDITOR Claire Cross

MANAGING ART EDITOR Philip Gilderdale

SENIOR ART EDITOR Karen Ward

ART EDITOR Glenda Fisher

DESIGNER Chloë Steers

PHOTOGRAPHY Steve Gorton and Andy Crawford

PRODUCTION Antony Heller

First published in Great Britain in 1997 by
Dorling Kindersley Limited,
9 Henrietta Street, London WC2E 8PS

8 10 9 7

A CIP catalogue record for this book is available from the British Library

ISBN 07513 03984

Reproduced by Bright Arts, Hong Kong
Printed and bound in China by L.Rex Printing Co., Ltd.

FOREWORD

During the past five to ten years, a bewildering number of new techniques have been introduced into the field of obstetrics and midwifery, all aimed at improving your prospects of having a normal, healthy baby. For example, ultrasound scanning, assisted conception techniques such as IVF, and major advances in the early diagnosis of genetic and chromosomal defects, are just a few of the discoveries that have revolutionized pregnancy care. At the same time, there has been a movement towards making pregnancy and childbirth a more natural and fulfilling experience for both mother and partner. Women are being offered different choices about the type of antenatal care they receive and where they should give birth.

All these issues and many more are explored in a simple question-and-answer format in this book. The authors are known to me personally to be a highly experienced team of two obstetricians and a midwife whose advice is both practical and professional. They have managed to communicate the more complex medical advances, and advice on more practical matters such as the preparations you need to make for birth whether in hospital or home, or choices for pain relief in labour, in a brilliantly clear and down-to-earth way.

I believe that this book will help you to make informed choices in your pregnancy in partnership with those looking after you and that this information will make your pregnancy a more enjoyable and rewarding experience.

Professor Stuart Campbell DSc FRCOG FRCPEd
DEPARTMENT OF OBSTETRICS AND GYNAECOLOGY
St George's Hospital
Tooting
London UK

FERTILITY AND CONCEPTION

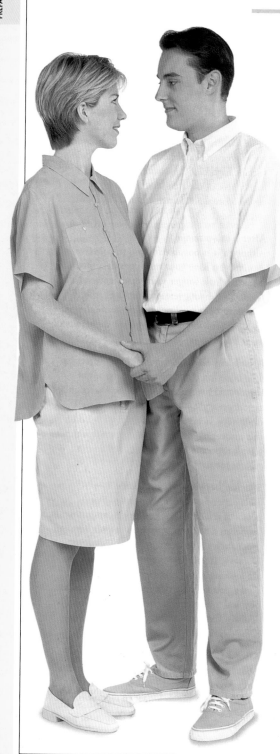

COMMON QUESTIONS ABOUT FERTILITY

QUESTIONS	ANSWERS
Will conception be difficult ...	
because I have painful or heavy periods?	Probably not, but if you have severe symptoms see your doctor to rule out an underlying cause such as fibroids, endometriosis or a pelvic infection.
because my periods are infrequent or irregular?	Possibly. Irregularity makes it harder to plan a pregnancy. You may need medical advice to work out whether you ovulate (see p. 12).
because both my partner and I are over 30?	Male fertility is not greatly affected by age, but the fertility of women over 35 does gradually decline.
because we both lead very busy, stressful lives, and hardly ever feel like making love?	Too much stress can put you off sex, and may also make your periods irregular. Regular exercise such as yoga and swimming, can help to relieve stress. If regular sex is unlikely, find out when you ovulate (see p. 12) and try to make love then.
because my partner had a sperm test and was told he had a low sperm count?	A low sperm count reduces a man's fertility and usually means that your partner needs special tests, and maybe treatment. There are several causes; simple treatment includes wearing looser underwear and reducing cigarettes and alcohol.
because I recently had a pelvic infection?	Severe or recurrent pelvic infections may lead to blocked or damaged Fallopian tubes (see opposite).

Q WHAT CAN REDUCE MY CHANCES OF CONCEPTION?

A Even if you are having sexual intercourse regularly, three main factors can reduce your chances of becoming pregnant: irregular or non-existent ovulation; damage to the Fallopian tubes; and reduced numbers of, or poor quality sperm. (See the panel, left, for other factors.)

Q WHEN SHOULD WE CONSULT A DOCTOR?

A Don't worry if you do not become pregnant at once. You have a 90 per cent chance of becoming pregnant within one year and a 95 per cent chance within two years. However, you should probably consult your doctor after trying for one year. If either of you suffers from a medical condition or if you are over 35 years old, ask for specialist advice earlier.

Q MY PARTNER IS GOING TO HAVE A SPERM TEST – WHAT IS THIS?

A If you have had problems conceiving, a sperm test will determine your partner's fertility. The sperm will be examined to see how well they move and how many abnormal sperm there are. The lower the proportion of healthy sperm, the more difficult it is to get pregnant, and the longer it may take.

Q MY FALLOPIAN TUBES ARE BLOCKED – DOES THIS MEAN I'M INFERTILE?

A The egg travels from the ovary to the womb through a Fallopian tube. This can be blocked or damaged by pelvic or abdominal infections, or an ectopic pregnancy (see p. 134), which reduce your chances of pregnancy.

Q WHEN ARE FERTILITY DRUGS USED?

A Fertility drugs are used when hormonal problems prevent ovulation (the release of eggs from the ovaries).

Q IF I TAKE FERTILITY DRUGS, WILL I HAVE TWINS OR MORE?

A Not necessarily, although the odds do increase; your chance of having twins is one in ten, compared to one in 90 for women who do not take fertility drugs.

Q WHAT OTHER OPTIONS ARE THERE TO HELP ME CONCEIVE?

A If simple treatments fail, options include surgery to unblock your Fallopian tubes, stronger fertility drugs, or your partner having treatment to improve his sperm count. If these fail, you may be offered assisted conception (see below).

WHAT IS ASSISTED CONCEPTION?

How is conception assisted?
Conception can be assisted by a number of methods including GIFT or IVF methods. GIFT (Gamete Intra-Fallopian Transfer) is a method whereby sperm and eggs are taken and mixed externally, then injected back into a Fallopian tube. IVF, which means In Vitro (in glass) Fertilization, involves eggs being removed and fertilized by sperm. As many as ten, or as few as three resultant embryos (fertilized eggs) are replaced in the womb. A new technique called ICSI (Intra Cytoplasmic Sperm Injection) injects sperm directly into the egg, and has revolutionized the treatment of male infertility.

When is assisted conception an option?
Assisted conception can be considered after a couple has been trying to conceive, without success, for several years, or when tests suggest that you are unlikely to become pregnant naturally.

What is the success rate?
The success rate varies widely depending on why you are having fertility treatment and the treatment you ultimately receive. One treatment cycle for IVF results in approximately a 25 per cent chance of pregnancy; with GIFT there is a 20 per cent chance. Becoming pregnant, unfortunately, does not guarantee "success" in the form of a healthy, term baby. Be sure to ask about both pregnancy and birth rates.

Will my pregnancy be any different from one that happens normally?
Medically, the pregnancy should be no different. However, you might be more worried about the chance of miscarriage, and inevitably, your emotional investment will be higher, especially if you see this as your last chance to have a child, or you feel that time is running out.

NOW THAT YOU'RE PREGNANT

Q I THINK I'M PREGNANT, HOW CAN I CONFIRM IT?

A There are three ways of confirming your pregnancy, by a urine test, a special blood test or occasionally an ultrasound scan. A urine test is the most common method by far and can be done at home with a pregnancy-testing kit, or you can take a urine sample to your doctor or to a family planning clinic and ask them to test it. A doctor's or clinic's test is usually free, but it takes a few days to get the results. Your doctor can also do a blood test, which detects pregnancy two weeks after conception. Although not a routine procedure, ultrasound can be used to confirm a pregnancy (particularly if you are not sure about your dates) but not for at least ten days after a missed period.

Q ARE HOME TEST KITS RELIABLE?

A If you follow the instructions carefully (see below), a home test kit is as accurate as a doctor's or family planning clinic's test. Its advantage is that it gives you an immediate answer; a sensitive testing kit can tell you that you are pregnant the day after your period is due.

Q WHAT ARE THE FIRST SIGNS OF PREGNANCY?

A A missed period is the most common sign of pregnancy but sometimes a period may not happen for other reasons, such as illness, shock or even jet lag. However, if you are experiencing other symptoms (see below), you should consider having a pregnancy test. Although not everybody feels the full range of symptoms as soon as they become pregnant, you may experience some of the following, which are most characteristic:

Signs of pregnancy
- You have missed one or more periods.
- You need to urinate frequently.
- You may find that certain tastes and smells become unpleasant suddenly; or you may crave odd foods. Often there may be a strange metallic taste in the mouth.
- You feel nauseous and may vomit in the mornings (or at other times of the day).
- Your breasts are tingling, tender or more swollen than usual.
- You feel particularly tired.
- You feel emotional or tearful.
- You suddenly become constipated.

HOW DO PREGNANCY TEST KITS WORK?

Pregnancy test kits require you to test a sample of your urine. The absorbent wand (below) reacts if a hormone called hCG (human chorionic gonadotrophin), which is produced by the embryo, is present in your urine. As a back-up, many kits include a second test.

Results windows   Cartridge   Absorbent pad

HOW TO USE A TEST KIT

Remove the test wand from the cap or cartridge. Hold the absorbent sampler in your urine stream for a few seconds. Replace the wand into the cartridge. Wait as directed. If you are pregnant, both windows will show a colour. (Not all kits look the same as the one shown here, but they work in the same way.).

Results windows

Pregnant   Not pregnant

Q WHAT SHOULD I DO WHEN MY PREGNANCY HAS BEEN CONFIRMED?

A It is a good idea to discuss your pregnancy with your doctor at the earliest opportunity. At this early stage, you need to have a check-up to ensure that all is going well, and to discuss how you want to organize your pregnancy care (see p. 22). If you are not registered with a doctor, you do need to contact a professional as soon as possible, preferably a doctor and/or a midwife, or otherwise visit your local hospital's antenatal clinic. If you would like to contact a midwife for advice, ask at your doctor's surgery about community midwives and which midwife schemes are available, or for names of local independent midwives (see p. 232).

Q WHY IS MY DOCTOR RECOMMENDING A SCAN TO CONFIRM MY DUE DATE?

A If your periods are irregular, you were on the Pill when you got pregnant, or you have a long cycle with infrequent periods, your doctor will find it more accurate to date your pregnancy by looking at the size of the baby on a scan.

Q I'VE MISSED MY PERIOD BUT THE TEST SHOWS NEGATIVE, WHAT DOES IT MEAN?

A The obvious answer is that your period may, for a variety of reasons, simply be late, or perhaps you haven't ovulated. Or you may be pregnant but your urine did not contain enough hCG (see box, opposite) to show on the test. Wait for a few days and try again.

WHEN IS MY BABY DUE?

If your periods are regular (about 28 days apart) and you have not been taking the Pill, your pregnancy is dated 40 weeks after the first day of your last menstrual period (LMP). There are several days around ovulation when fertilization could have taken place, so pregnancy is not dated from the time of fertility or sexual intercourse. You will be considered four weeks pregnant when you miss your first period.

HOW TO USE THE CHART

Look up the first day of your last period in the light-coloured line next to the months that are in heavy type. The figure below it will be the estimated date of your delivery (EDD). For example, if your last period began on April 15, you will see that your EDD is January 20. In a leap year add one day to any date after February 29.

	1	2	3	4	5	6	7	8	9	10	11	12	13	14	15	16	17	18	19	20	21	22	23	24	25	26	27	28	29	30	31
JANUARY	1	2	3	4	5	6	7	8	9	10	11	12	13	14	15	16	17	18	19	20	21	22	23	24	25	26	27	28	29	30	31
OCT/NOV	8	9	10	11	12	13	14	15	16	17	18	19	20	21	22	23	24	25	26	27	28	29	30	31	1	2	3	4	5	6	7
FEBRUARY	1	2	3	4	5	6	7	8	9	10	11	12	13	14	15	16	17	18	19	20	21	22	23	24	25	26	27	28			
NOV/DEC	8	9	10	11	12	13	14	15	16	17	18	19	20	21	22	23	24	25	26	27	28	29	30	1	2	3	4	5			
MARCH	1	2	3	4	5	6	7	8	9	10	11	12	13	14	15	16	17	18	19	20	21	22	23	24	25	26	27	28	29	30	31
DEC/JAN	6	7	8	9	10	11	12	13	14	15	16	17	18	19	20	21	22	23	24	25	26	27	28	29	30	31	1	2	3	4	5
APRIL	1	2	3	4	5	6	7	8	9	10	11	12	13	14	15	16	17	18	19	20	21	22	23	24	25	26	27	28	29	30	
JAN/FEB	6	7	8	9	10	11	12	13	14	15	16	17	18	19	20	21	22	23	24	25	26	27	28	29	30	31	1	2	3	4	
MAY	1	2	3	4	5	6	7	8	9	10	11	12	13	14	15	16	17	18	19	20	21	22	23	24	25	26	27	28	29	30	31
FEB/MARCH	5	6	7	8	9	10	11	12	13	14	15	16	17	18	19	20	21	22	23	24	25	26	27	28	1	2	3	4	5	6	7
JUNE	1	2	3	4	5	6	7	8	9	10	11	12	13	14	15	16	17	18	19	20	21	22	23	24	25	26	27	28	29	30	
MARCH/APRIL	8	9	10	11	12	13	14	15	16	17	18	19	20	21	22	23	24	25	26	27	28	29	30	31	1	2	3	4	5	6	
JULY	1	2	3	4	5	6	7	8	9	10	11	12	13	14	15	16	17	18	19	20	21	22	23	24	25	26	27	28	29	30	31
APRIL/MAY	7	8	9	10	11	12	13	14	15	16	17	18	19	20	21	22	23	24	25	26	27	28	29	30	1	2	3	4	5	6	7
AUGUST	1	2	3	4	5	6	7	8	9	10	11	12	13	14	15	16	17	18	19	20	21	22	23	24	25	26	27	28	29	30	31
MAY/JUNE	8	9	10	11	12	13	14	15	16	17	18	19	20	21	22	23	24	25	26	27	28	29	30	31	1	2	3	4	5	6	7
SEPTEMBER	1	2	3	4	5	6	7	8	9	10	11	12	13	14	15	16	17	18	19	20	21	22	23	24	25	26	27	28	29	30	
JUNE/JULY	8	9	10	11	12	13	14	15	16	17	18	19	20	21	22	23	24	25	26	27	28	29	30	1	2	3	4	5	6	7	
OCTOBER	1	2	3	4	5	6	7	8	9	10	11	12	13	14	15	16	17	18	19	20	21	22	23	24	25	26	27	28	29	30	31
JULY/AUGUST	8	9	10	11	12	13	14	15	16	17	18	19	20	21	22	23	24	25	26	27	28	29	30	31	1	2	3	4	5	6	7
NOVEMBER	1	2	3	4	5	6	7	8	9	10	11	12	13	14	15	16	17	18	19	20	21	22	23	24	25	26	27	28	29	30	
AUGUST/SEPT	8	9	10	11	12	13	14	15	16	17	18	19	20	21	22	23	24	25	26	27	28	29	30	31	1	2	3	4	5	6	
DECEMBER	1	2	3	4	5	6	7	8	9	10	11	12	13	14	15	16	17	18	19	20	21	22	23	24	25	26	27	28	29	30	31
SEPT/OCT	7	8	9	10	11	12	13	14	15	16	17	18	19	20	21	22	23	24	25	26	27	28	29	30	1	2	3	4	5	6	7

CONCERNS IN EARLY PREGNANCY

Q WE'VE LONGED FOR THIS BABY, SO WHY AM I UPSET AND CONFUSED?

A Give yourself time to adjust to the idea of being pregnant. It is not unusual to feel confused, or to feel ecstatic one minute and scared the next. Once you accept that the coming baby is a reality, you should be able to enjoy your pregnancy to the full.

Q I DRANK ALCOHOL BEFORE I KNEW I WAS PREGNANT, IS THIS BAD FOR MY BABY?

A Although regular, excessive drinking during pregnancy is bad for your baby, the likelihood of your baby being affected by a little over-indulgence in early pregnancy is very small. Whether you are planning a pregnancy or have recently discovered that you are pregnant, it is always best to avoid alcohol.

Q MY CERVICAL SMEAR TEST INDICATED AN ABNORMALITY, IS IT IMPORTANT?

A There are different degrees of seriousness in smear abnormalities. However, irrespective of the degree of the abnormality, it is unlikely that you will need or be given treatment for this while you are pregnant. Nevertheless, even though treatment for abnormal smears is unusual during pregnancy, you should not ignore any smear abnormality and it is best to seek medical advice from your doctor.

Q I HAVE HAD TREATMENT TO MY CERVIX – WILL THIS AFFECT MY PREGNANCY?

A Modern treatments for an abnormal smear are very unlikely to affect your pregnancy but if you have had treatment to your cervix, you should mention this to your doctor at your first antenatal visit. Also, if you have had a cone biopsy (the removal of a cone-shaped area of cervical tissue), there is a slightly increased risk of having a late miscarriage or of a premature labour. Most women have normal pregnancies after cone biopsies.

Q DO I NEED GENETIC COUNSELLING?

A You may need advice if you are over the age of 35; if you or your partner have or are carriers of a genetic or chromosome disorder; if you have previously had a child with a chromosomal or genetic problem; or tests have shown problems in the baby you are carrying (see p. 34).

Q WILL MY SECOND PREGNANCY BE LIKE MY FIRST?

A In general, no two pregnancies are the same. Many women find that subsequent pregnancies are physically and psychologically easier than their first. To some extent this is because you are more aware of what to expect. Physical symptoms of early pregnancy, such as nausea and vomiting, are sometimes less severe.

I HAVE DISCOVERED THAT I AM PREGNANT ACCIDENTALLY...

... while taking the Pill. Will this have affected the baby?
The hormones in the Pill (both the combined oral contraceptive and the Mini-pill) are similar to the oestrogen and progesterone that occur naturally in your body. The amount of hormones in the Pill is very small and once you stop taking it the hormones will disappear very rapidly from your body, so it is very unlikely to cause any harm to the developing baby.

...while I have a coil in place. Should it be removed?
It is important to establish first that the pregnancy is in the womb rather than in a Fallopian tube; this can be established by an ultrasound scan. If the pregnancy is at an early stage, the coil is usually removed but there is a small risk of miscarriage. It is more difficult to remove the coil later on; it may be left where it is, and the baby is usually born unharmed.

... after taking the morning-after pill. Has this harmed the pregnancy?
There is no evidence that the morning-after pill has caused abnormalities in any babies. However, if only to set your mind at rest, you could go back to the clinic where you got the pill, have the pregnancy confirmed, and discuss any possible ill-effects, as well as whether a termination of the pregnancy is advisable.

WHAT COULD HARM MY BABY?

	RISK TO BABY	ADVICE
Alcohol	Your baby's development can be harmed by alcohol because alcohol crosses the placenta and enters into your baby's bloodstream.	It is probably best to avoid any alcohol in the first trimester. Binge drinking can be particularly harmful (see p. 103).
Animals and pet litter	Toxoplasma infection, which may cause blindness, mental retardation, and deafness (see p. 30).	Avoid direct skin contact with cat litter and use gloves while gardening.
Chemicals: hair dyes, permanents; chlorine in pools	There is no evidence of any harm.	There is no reason to avoid swimming pools. Follow the manufacturer's instructions when using dyes.
Cigarettes	Smoking more than ten cigarettes a day can reduce your baby's birth weight and cause problems during pregnancy, labour, and your baby's first weeks of life (see p. 102).	Smoking should be stopped completely during pregnancy – not only does it affect the blood supply to the womb and oxygen to the baby, it also harms the mother's lungs and circulation.
Particular foods	Listeria bacteria found in some foods can cause miscarriage or stillbirth. Excess Vitamin A may cause birth defects. Salmonella can cause miscarriage.	Avoid pâtés and unpasteurized dairy products such as soft cheeses. Avoid all undercooked meats and offal, especially pork, as well as raw fish (sushi). Do not eat liver or liver pâté. Avoid raw or partially cooked eggs (see p. 102).
Infectious illnesses	Chickenpox, mumps, and measles are all potentially harmful to the developing baby (see p. 121). German measles (rubella) may cause severe abnormalities, but most women are vaccinated against this.	Avoid contact with young children who may have an infection. Contracting rubella may be a reason to consider termination. If you are worried, talk to your doctor.
	Genital herpes may cause severe infection in the baby after delivery.	Contact your doctor if you have herpes or develop genital blisters or ulcers (see p. 120).
Strenuous physical activity	Exercise in moderation will not harm you or your pregnancy.	It is sensible to avoid heavy lifting and any activity that involves the risk of injury. Don't take up any new strenuous physical activity.
Stress	There is no evidence of any harm.	Avoid becoming very stressed because it will add to your fatigue. It may also reduce your enjoyment of your pregnancy.
VDUs, microwaves, and photocopiers	There is no evidence of any harm.	Use them as you would normally.
X-rays	It is possible that X-rays during the first 13 weeks may harm the development of your baby's main organ systems.	X-rays (including dental ones) aren't usually done in the first 13 weeks. If an X-ray is necessary, make sure your doctor or X-ray technician knows you are pregnant, so that a low dose of X-rays will be used.

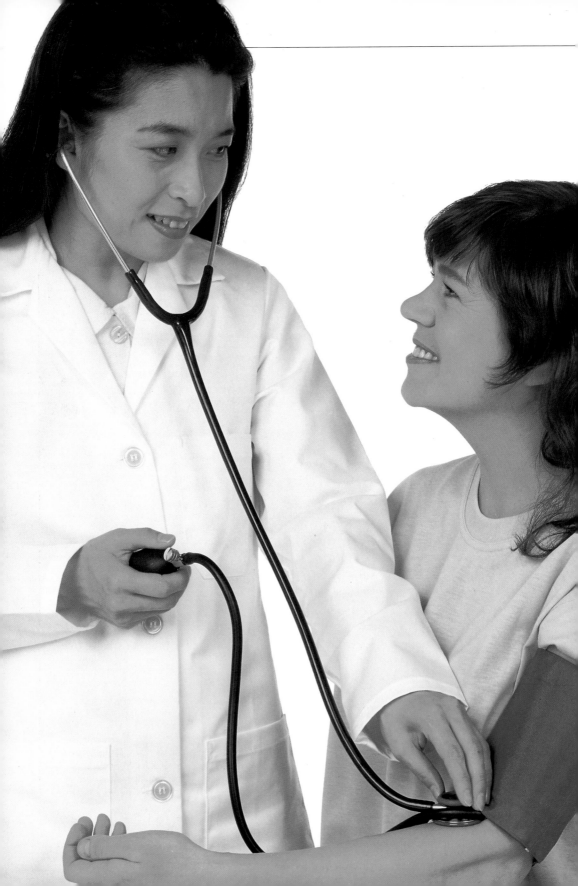

YOUR ANTENATAL CARE

Now that you know that you are pregnant, you will want to find out as much as possible about your physical condition, what to expect in the coming months, and what plans you should be making for your labour. This chapter provides detailed information about the antenatal tests you may have, as well as your choices in antenatal care and labour so that you can decide what would suit you and your partner. Whether you would prefer a home birth or a hospital birth, these options are discussed. It also explains where you could have your antenatal care, who your professional carers are likely to be, and what happens at your first check-up.

ANTENATAL VISITS

Q HOW OFTEN DO I HAVE CHECK-UPS?

A The first and longest check-up is the "booking" visit, between the eighth and twelfth week of your pregnancy. Routine check-ups are at monthly intervals thereafter until 28 weeks, then every other week until 36 weeks; finally, they are once a week until your delivery. You may need more check-ups if you are expecting twins or if a complication develops, and fewer if you are low-risk (see p. 28). If necessary, you can contact the clinic between visits.

Q DO I HAVE TO ATTEND EVERY APPOINTMENT?

A Antenatal care is a service that is offered to ensure the well-being of you and your baby. You may have to miss a visit for unavoidable reasons but this is unlikely to cause harm. It is, however, best to attend even if you feel well.

Q CAN MY PARTNER COME WITH ME?

A Yes, if he is able to, it is a good idea. During the first visit, he can answer questions about his medical history and that of his family; he can ask any questions, and see what happens when you have check-ups. Perhaps most importantly, your partner will feel more involved with his baby if he shares in the pregnancy process.

Q DO I NEED TO DO ANYTHING BEFORE MY FIRST VISIT?

A You may find it helpful to read any leaflets or information that the hospital has sent you. Check if there are any inherited abnormalities or diseases in either family. Make a note of the date of your last period, and the dates of any previous pregnancies and/or miscarriages. Think about and write down any questions you wish to ask.

WHAT DO THE NOTES ON MY ANTENATAL RECORD MEAN?

When you attend your first antenatal check-up you will be given a wallet or a page of notes. Bring your notes to every appointment because they contain personal details such as your blood group. Your doctor or midwife will fill in information on your progress; certain abbreviations are always used by them (see below).

BP Your blood pressure.
NAD Nothing abnormal detected, usually in your urine.
Hb Haemoglobin levels that indicate anaemia if low.
Fe Iron tablets.
FHH/NH Fetal heart heard or not heard, usually from about 14 weeks. Also FHHR, which means fetal heart heard and regular.
FMF Fetal movements felt, usually from 16–20 weeks.
Ceph Cephalic, means baby is head down in the womb.
Vx Vertex, also means baby is head down.

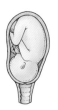

Cephalic or vertex   Breech

Br Breech. Your baby is bottom down in the womb.
Eng/E Engaged. The baby's head has dropped into the pelvic cavity ready for delivery.
NE Not engaged (see above).
SFH Symphysis fundal height is the measurement of the length of the womb (in centimetres)

from the top of the pubic bone, and indicates the growth of the pregnancy.
PP Presenting part, which refers to that part of the baby that is lying lowest.
Primagravida A woman who is in her first pregnancy.
Multigravida A woman who has been pregnant before.
EDD Estimated date of delivery.
Oed Oedema, which means swelling of the hands, feet, and face.
CS/LSCS Caesarean section or lower segment Caesarean section.
TCA To come again.

Q WHO WILL I SEE AT MY FIRST ANTENATAL APPOINTMENT?

A At the hospital a midwife usually handles the history-taking and tests before passing you on to an obstetrician who will carry out a physical (and possibly an internal) examination. Should there be any complications, you may also have to see the consultant obstetrician. If you have opted for the Domino or Team system (see p. 23), this check-up is carried out by a midwife in your home, and lasts about 1½ hours.

Q WHAT HAPPENS AT LATER ANTENATAL APPOINTMENTS?

A The checks-ups at later appointments are less comprehensive and therefore shorter. There are several procedures that are routinely carried out at each check-up. Your weight is noted, your urine tested, and your blood pressure checked. Your baby's position and stage of growth are established and the heartbeat heard. You will be asked about your baby's movements. Blood tests are taken at intervals or if you are having special investigations.

WHO ARE THE PROFESSIONAL CARERS?

During your pregnancy, labour, and after the birth, you will meet a number of health professionals who will give the advice and care that you and your baby need. Your doctor or midwife will probably be the professionals you see most often; at most check-ups you may not necessarily see anyone other than a midwife. Usually you will need to speak to a consultant obstetrician only if you have a problem and, (apart from the first check-up) to a paediatrician only if your baby has one.

Doctor, general practitioner (GP)
Your doctor has a pivotal role during your pregnancy. He/she is also your first point of contact when you wish to find out about your pregnancy and your options. Usually, those looking after you and your baby will refer back to your doctor's initial contact and notes. Your doctor books the hospital or writes to the community midwife for you once you have decided where you wish to go to have your baby. Doctors sometimes have their own antenatal clinics or GP units. Some doctors are able to be involved with the delivery itself but if this is not feasible, he/she will visit you afterwards at home.

Midwife
A midwife is trained in the speciality of childbirth and is responsible for providing care in normal pregnancies. She (and it is usually but not always a woman) is recognized as an independent practitioner and may work within a hospital, in the community or both. Her role includes caring for you and your baby before, during and after the birth, either at home or in hospital, provided that all goes well. If there should be any complication, it is the midwife's role to work alongside the obstetricians to provide the appropriate care. A midwife is an excellent source of practical advice on pregnancy, birth, and baby care as well as of more technical medical information.

Obstetrician
This is a doctor who has trained as a specialist in the care of pregnant women and after many years and a wealth of experience will become a consultant obstetrician.

Consultant obstetrician
The most senior doctor in the obstetrics department, as head of the team of doctors looking after you, the consultant has the final say if there are any problems. His/her name will also appear on your personal notes. Consultants are experts in the complications of pregnancy, so you will probably have little contact with them if your pregnancy is problem-free. However, you have a right to speak with your consultant at any stage of your pregnancy should you wish.

Paediatrician
A doctor who specializes in the health of babies and children, a paediatrican attends all "abnormal" deliveries and multiple births, or when the baby is delivered with forceps, or by Caesarean section. All newborn babies are checked by a paediatrician before they go home.

Health visitor
A health visitor has had specialist training in family health and is often an ex-nurse or midwife. She will contact you before and after the delivery.

ANTENATAL MONITORING

Q HOW IS IT DECIDED WHETHER MY PREGNANCY IS LOW- OR HIGH-RISK?

A There are certain factors that constitute a risk to you and/or your baby. Some of these you can do something about, such as stopping smoking or not taking street drugs. Other factors, such as twins or a large baby, you can do nothing about. However, by careful antenatal monitoring the likelihood of unexpected complications is reduced; should something unforeseen happen, your professional carers will be prepared. In pregnancy care there is an adage that "the best predictor of the future is the past"; this means that if you had a problem in a previous pregnancy, the same problem may recur.

General risks that may affect your pregnancy
- Alcohol abuse.
- Smoking.
- You are very thin or very large.
- You have a restrictive diet or are malnourished.
- You take street drugs such as heroin or cocaine.
- You have a medical condition requiring drugs.

Risks that mean you need close antenatal care
- Previous pre-term delivery (before 37 weeks).
- Baby in previous pregnancy had an abnormality.
- You have diabetes and/or high blood pressure.
- Previous thrombosis (blood clot).

Risks that mean you need extra care in your delivery
- Very large baby (estimated weight over 4kg/8½lb).
- Very small baby (estimated weight less than 2.5kg/5½lb).
- Twins.
- Breech baby.
- A previous delivery by Caesarean section.
- Previous problems in delivery such as haemorrhage (excessive bleeding).
- High blood pressure in pregnancy (pre-eclampsia).
- Diabetes.

Low-risk pregnancies
If none of the risks listed above applies to you, and any previous pregnancy and delivery were normal and uneventful, it is unlikely that you will have a problem that needs special care. It is nevertheless essential to attend all your antenatal appointments so that your health and the health of your baby can be regularly monitored.

WHAT DO THE ROUTINE BLOOD TESTS SHOW?

■ **Your blood group and Rhesus (Rh) status**
It is important for your doctor to know which blood group you belong to in case you need a blood transfusion during the pregnancy or labour. The most common is group O; A, B, and AB are much less common. Your Rhesus status is either positive or negative, so that you may be O negative or A positive and so on. Rhesus positive simply means that there is a special identifying label on your blood cells, which is not there if you are Rhesus negative. If you are Rhesus negative, a further test will be done to check if any antibodies are present; the tests will be repeated at intervals during your pregnancy. If there are antibodies present, your partner will also need to give blood for testing.

■ **Your haemoglobin (red blood cells) levels**
Red cells contain iron and carry oxygen; if the test shows that the level of red cells is low, you are anaemic, and you will be advised to eat foods with a high iron content, or you may have to take iron tablets. Anaemia can cause you to feel very tired (see p. 125) and it will also be a problem if you bleed during your pregnancy or at delivery.

■ **Rubella (German measles)** A blood test shows whether you are immune to the disease. If you aren't, you could contract rubella in early pregnancy; this could cause blindness, deafness, and heart defects in your baby (see p. 121).

■ **Syphilis** Because it is now so easily cured, this sexually transmitted disease is rare these days. However, if the disease is present and untreated in pregnancy, it could cause the baby to have congenital and developmental problems.

■ **Hepatitis B** This liver disease, caused by a virus, can be passed to the baby and cause serious liver damage in the baby.

■ **Other blood tests** You may be offered other blood tests (see p. 30).

SPECIAL INVESTIGATIONS

Q WHY MIGHT I NEED SPECIAL INVESTIGATIONS?

A You will normally be offered further tests if there is a significant reason to suspect your baby might be suffering from a disease or an abnormality. The decision may be made on the basis of your age (over 35); if your routine scan (see p. 32) shows a problem; if you and/or your partner suffer from a hereditary disease; or if you have previously had a baby with an abnormality.

Q WHAT TESTS WILL I HAVE?

A There are several sorts of tests which detect or rule out problems. Initially, tests on your blood may detect problems in the baby such as Down's syndrome or spina bifida (see Triple Test, p. 30), or a problem you may have, such as diabetes. An ultrasound scan may reassure you that the baby seems to be normal and is growing well; it will also reveal any major defects. If the blood tests or scan do detect a problem, then further tests such as amniocentesis may be offered: this involves taking a sample of fluid from inside the womb (see p. 36).

Q WHAT ABNORMALITIES CAN BE DETECTED?

A There are three kinds of abnormalities that occur: congenital, chromosomal, and genetic. Congenital abnormalities can usually be detected on an ultrasound scan at 18 to 22 weeks (see p. 32). Chromosomal and genetic abnormalities are detected by invasive tests such as amniocentesis, cordocentesis, and CVS (see p. 36).

Q WHAT ARE CONGENITAL ABNORMALITIES?

A This term means that the baby has developed a physical abnormality, such as hare lip, heart and brain defects, spina bifida, absent limbs or extra digits, in the womb. There is no genetic or chromosomal reason for this and often no cause whatsoever is found; it happens rarely when, for instance, the mother contracts an infection such as rubella (German measles). Congenital abnormalities can also be the result of dietary imbalances (such as a lack of folic acid), or because a harmful drug was taken in early pregnancy.

Q WHAT HAPPENS IF A CONGENITAL ABNORMALITY IS DISCOVERED?

A The less severe abnormalities such as hare lip, club foot, and extra digits can usually be dealt with surgically after the baby is born; often the baby is otherwise completely normal. Severe abnormalities such as major heart and central nervous system (brain and spinal cord) malformations often result in miscarriage or death of the baby before 24 weeks. In either situation you will be referred to a consultant to discuss all the options.

DISCUSSION POINT

DO I HAVE TO HAVE SPECIAL TESTS?

The most difficult aspect of medical intervention is that it tells you facts about your pregnancy that you might have preferred not to know, and you may not wish to proceed with further tests.

Positive results

There is little point in having screening for any abnormality unless you have carefully thought through what you would do if the results were positive. Once you know there is a problem, and realize the severity of the condition, you will have to decide whether to continue with the pregnancy or not.

Difficult decisions

Whether to terminate the pregnancy on the basis of what tests show is a question about which medical and popular opinion is divided. Some couples want only a completely "normal" baby and so would wish to have a termination. Others are prepared to continue with the pregnancy and raise a child with special needs; some cannot consider a termination. Knowing how you feel about this issue will help you and your medical advisors should a difficult decision be necessary.

SPECIAL BLOOD TESTS

Q WHY MIGHT I NEED SPECIAL BLOOD TESTS?

A Special blood tests are the tools of diagnosis. There are three types of tests: the tests that detect existing diseases that might affect the pregnancy – these include diabetes and HIV; the tests that detect problem genes that you may be unaware of but could pass on to the baby – these include tests for thalassaemia and sickle cell anaemia (see below); tests that measure substances in your blood that indicate possible fetal abnormalities, and these include the Triple or Bart's test, which tests for Down's syndrome.

Q DOES THE TRIPLE BLOOD TEST GIVE A DEFINITE ANSWER?

A The Triple or Bart's test is a screening test, which means that the result of the test is not absolute, but an indication of the risk of your baby being affected. Carried out at 15 to 16 weeks, along with an ultrasound scan, this test is based on the level of hormones in your blood. Usually, if the test shows that the risk of your baby having Down's syndrome is greater than 1 in 270, you will be offered an invasive test, such as amniocentesis or cordocentesis, to confirm or deny that the baby is free of this condition (see p. 36).

WHAT ARE THE SPECIAL BLOOD TESTS?

TEST	WHO IS TESTED	WHAT IT TESTS FOR
Triple or Bart's test (for Down's syndrome, see above)	Depends on local policy but it is usually offered to women over the age of 35 or those with a higher risk of a Down's baby.	It shows the level of three substances that are found in the blood stream of the mother: alpha-fetoprotein (AFP), oestriol, and human chorionic gonadotrophin (hCG).
Glucose tolerance test (for diabetes)	Women at risk of diabetes include those who are known to have high blood sugar, sugar in the urine, diabetes in a previous pregnancy, or a large baby.	After a sugary drink, four samples of blood are taken over the next two hours. If your blood sugar level remains high, this can indicate the presence of diabetes.
HIV test (for human immunodeficiency virus)	Anyone who is at risk may ask to be tested. This is done only with your consent.*	It detects the presence of antibodies for the HIV virus.
Sickle cell test (for sickle cell anaemia)	If you, or any of your ancestors, originate from an area where this trait is widespread, especially Africa and the West Indies.	It looks at the type of haemoglobin in your red blood cells and detects the sickle cells.
Haemoglobin electrophoresis test for thalassaemia	If you, or any of your ancestors, originate from an area where this trait is widespread, especially Asia and parts of Africa.	It identifies in red blood cells the different haemoglobins that denote thalassaemia disease.
Toxoplasmosis test	If you have had a recent flu-like illness, especially if you have been in contact with pets and farm animals.	It looks for antibodies to toxoplasma in your blood, which suggest that you have been infected.

*Anonymous HIV testing is carried out on blood samples in many hospitals. No samples are named and the result cannot be traced to you. If you want a "named" test, you will be offered counselling.

Q WHEN DO I NEED TO HAVE THE TEST FOR TOXOPLASMOSIS?

A Toxoplasmosis is a parasitic disease that is passed on to humans by domestic cats, and, more rarely, by sheep and pigs. If this disease is contracted during pregnancy, toxoplasma can cross the placenta and cause blindness, epilepsy, and learning difficulties in the baby. A blood test indicates whether or not you are immune to this disease. You will not usually be offered this test unless there is a high risk that you have been exposed to the illness. If the test shows you have contracted the disease, you may need an ultrasound scan to discover if the baby's growth has been affected. In the UK only about 20 per cent of women are immune to this disease.

WHAT HAPPENS IF A TEST IS POSITIVE

This test screens only. If it is positive you have an increased risk of having a Down's baby. To diagnose this absolutely, you need a further invasive test such as an amniocentesis or cordocentesis (see p. 36).

You are treated for diabetes, which means close control of your diet, possibly with insulin injections as well, and extra antenatal check-ups. You may also have to have more than the average two ultrasound scans.

Any infections that you develop must be carefully treated. The risk of transmitting HIV to the baby can be reduced by certain measures at delivery (see p. 124).

If sickle cell trait or disease is detected, your partner should be tested as well. If he is positive, the baby is at risk of being born with the disease. An amniocentesis or cordocentesis test will confirm this (see p. 36).

If this trait is detected, the baby may develop the disease. Also, you may become anaemic and require iron and folic acid supplements.

You may need to have antibiotics to treat the baby, and ultrasound scans to see if the baby's growth is being affected by the illness (see p. 32).

Q MY DOCTOR WANTS TO TEST ME FOR DIABETES, WHY?

A Your doctor is probably suggesting this because sugar has been found in your urine after several tests, your blood sugar level is high, or you are carrying a large baby – all may indicate diabetes.

Q WHY IS UNTREATED DIABETES A PROBLEM IN PREGNANCY?

A Diabetes occurs when your body is not producing sufficient insulin for its needs. When diabetes develops because of the demands of pregnancy on your body, it is called "gestational diabetes", which is not usually as serious as pre-existing diabetes (see p. 125). Insulin is essential for regulating sugar conversion and for the metabolism of fats and protein. If diabetes is not correctly treated by a carefully controlled diet or regular insulin, this condition can make you feel thirsty, weak, and very unwell, and may cause problems for the baby.

Q I HAD DIABETES IN MY LAST PREGNANCY, WILL I GET IT AGAIN?

A If you developed diabetes in a previous pregnancy, even if it subsequently got better after the delivery of your baby, you have a higher chance of developing it again. This means you will automatically be given an extra blood test for glucose between 20 to 26 weeks, or a "glucose tolerance test" (see chart, left).

Q WHEN SHOULD I HAVE AN HIV TEST?

A HIV stands for Human Immunodeficiency Virus. It is a "retrovirus", which means that it incorporates itself into the genetic material of the cells in your body, especially those white blood cells that are important for fighting infections. There is as yet no known cure. You should think about having a test if you or your partner are from an area such as Central Africa and parts of Asia where HIV is prevalent; if your partner past or present was a possible carrier of HIV; or if you have injected drugs and shared needles.

Q IF I AM HIV POSITIVE, WILL IT AFFECT MY BABY?

A If you are otherwise well, your pregnancy will not necessarily be affected. However, the disease can be transmitted to the baby but there are ways of reducing this risk at or after delivery. Some women opt for a termination.

DOPPLER AND NUCHAL SCANS

Q **WHAT ARE THESE SCANS FOR?**

A Doppler and Nuchal scans are both painless and non-invasive special ultrasound scans that are used to detect specific problems. Both types of scan are relatively new and they are available only at certain hospitals.

Q **WHEN IS A DOPPLER SCAN OFFERED?**

A A Doppler scan is used to examine the blood flow in the baby or in the placenta. It is used to check babies who are small in relation to their due date or not growing as fast as expected. The test may also identify women at risk of developing high blood pressure (pre-eclampsia), (see p. 127).

Q **HOW DOES A DOPPLER SCAN WORK?**

A It uses a different form of high-frequency sound waves, which are processed to show special wave forms. These sound waves reflect off moving objects, particularly red blood cells moving through arteries and veins. A Doppler scan shows the speed at which these cells are travelling; this tells doctors about the flow of blood through the blood vessels, indicates whether the placenta is working properly, or if the baby is short of oxygen.

Q **IS A DOPPLER SCAN SAFE?**

A The Doppler scan has been used in obstetrics, gynaecology, and many other areas of medicine for at least ten years and it has never caused any safety concerns. However, to be on the safe side, it is not used in very early pregnancy. It tends to be available only at larger hospitals with specialist units.

Q **WHAT IS A NUCHAL SCAN AND IS IT SAFE?**

A A Nuchal scan is an ultrasound scan in which the baby's neck is examined (see below). It is a fairly new but safe method of early antenatal screening for Down's syndrome. Although it does not give a definitive answer, it can show at a very early stage if there is a chance that your baby has Down's. It may be the best non-invasive test available at the moment. If it shows this risk is high, you can be offered amniocentesis or CVS (see p. 36).

WHAT DOES A NUCHAL SCAN SHOW?

"Nuchal" means neck; Nuchal ultrasound scan, carried out at 11 to 14 weeks, is used to look at the thickness of the baby's neck. It is thought that babies with a particularly thick nuchal pad at the back of the neck are at higher risk of suffering from heart defects, Down's syndrome, or some other chromosomal problem. If it appears that your baby has a thicker nuchal pad, you will be offered a subsequent amniocentesis or other invasive test (see p. 36) to confirm, or rule out, these problems.

WHAT THE SCAN SHOWS
The picture (right) shows the scan of a normal baby. The dotted lines indicate where the nuchal pad would be thicker in a Down's syndrome baby. The baby's neck is measured between the points indicated; if the nuchal pad is larger than normal, chromosomal problems or heart defects are more likely.

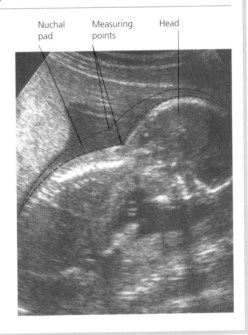

Nuchal pad   Measuring points   Head

CONFIRMING THE DIAGNOSIS

Q HOW IS A DIAGNOSIS CONFIRMED?

A If, as a result of what the special blood tests and/or the ultrasound scans show, there is reason to suspect that your baby may be suffering from a disease, or a genetic or chromosomal abnormality, further invasive tests will be suggested (see p. 36) to confirm, or rule out, these problems.

Q WHAT ARE GENETIC ABNORMALITIES?

A Genetic abnormalities are those diseases that occur usually because of a defective gene that you or your partner is carrying, but do not necessarily know that you possess.

Q WHAT ARE GENETIC DISEASES?

A Examples of these are: cystic fibrosis, a rare disease of the lungs and digestive systems that occurs in around 1 in 2,000 pregnancies; sickle cell anaemia and thalassaemia, which are common in certain ethnic groups. Babies suffering from these conditions are usually perfectly well in the womb and the illness only shows itself after birth. There are also some sex-linked conditions, such as muscular dystrophy and haemophilia, that are carried by the mother and passed to male children; you will almost certainly know if you have these genes in your family.

Q HOW MIGHT MY BABY HAVE A GENETIC DISEASE IF I DON'T HAVE ANY DISEASES?

A The genes for some diseases are recessive, or hidden. If both parents have the same gene, the two sets of genes may match up in your baby, which means that your baby will suffer from the full condition. Some genes are passed directly from one or other parent. Occasionally, diseases occur due to a spontaneous mutation of the genes.

Q WHAT ARE CHROMOSOMAL ABNORMALITIES?

A Chromosomal abnormalities include Down's syndrome and other, usually fatal but very rare, chromosomal syndromes. In Down's syndrome an extra chromosome 21 is present, which results in a child with physical abnormalities and learning difficulties (see p. 132). It occurs more frequently in babies of older mothers (see right).

HOW LIKELY IS IT THAT MY BABY WILL HAVE DOWN'S SYNDROME?

The risk of having a baby with Down's syndrome is related to your age, although parents of any age can have a Down's child; it is not related to how many children you have had, whether you have a new partner, nor to any drugs that you might have taken at or around conception.

YOUR RISK INCREASE

IN YOUR TWENTIES
You have a 1 in 1,000 chance.

IN YOUR THIRTIES
You have a 1 in 900 chance. At 35, this increases to 1 in 400. At 37, it becomes 1 in 250.

IN YOUR FORTIES
You begin with a 1 in 100 chance and by the time you are 45 it has increased to 1 in 25.

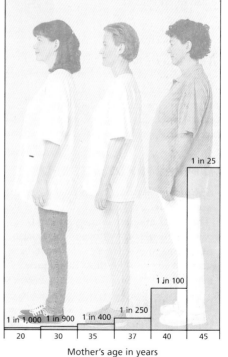

| 1 in 1,000 | 1 in 900 | 1 in 400 | 1 in 250 | 1 in 100 | 1 in 25 |

| 20 | 30 | 35 | 37 | 40 | 45 |

Mother's age in years

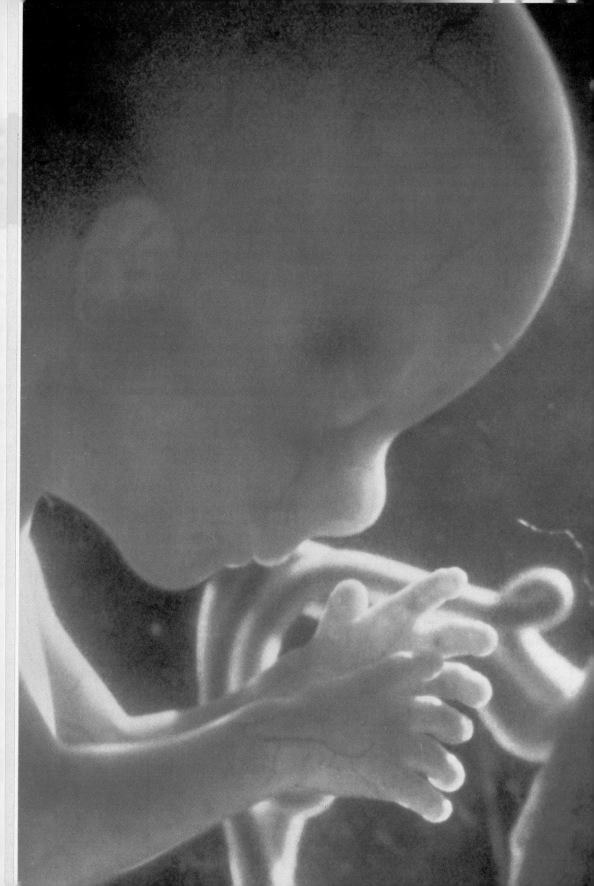

YOUR
DEVELOPING
BABY

Inside your expanding womb your baby is
growing, taking from you all the nourishment
he or she needs to become a unique human
being. What started as a microscopic two-celled
egg will, by only 12 weeks, have developed into
a tiny but perfectly formed baby. Although, at
this stage, you cannot detect any movements, as
the weeks pass you will be able to feel his or
her presence in your body. This chapter
explores the miracle of this new life in detail,
showing exactly how your baby develops from
conception to term – month-by-month – and
giving you a complete and fascinating picture
of what is happening to you and your baby.

HOW YOUR BABY GROWS

AT THE MOMENT OF conception, when the sperm penetrates the egg, the genes from both parents join to make a new combination, and your child, a unique human being, is created. Below is a visual summary of this miraculous achievement. Your pregnancy is looked at in three stages. The first 12 weeks – the first trimester – are crucial for your baby's development. Although you may not be aware of it, the cluster of cells is multiplying into a fully formed (but immature) human being.

From 13 to 25 weeks – the second trimester – your baby grows rapidly, about 5cm (2in) a month, and can now make facial expressions, swallow, hear, and kick. By 26 weeks – the third trimester – your baby could survive if born. In the last three months, he or she should double in weight, weighing an average 3.4kg (7lb 7oz) at birth.

STAGES OF DEVELOPMENT

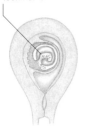

The fetus begins to look human

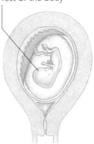

The head grows faster than the rest of the body

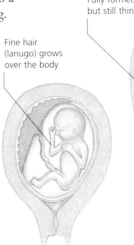

Fine hair (lanugo) grows over the body

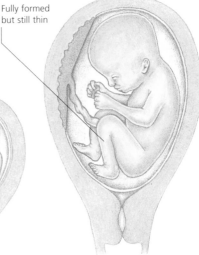

Fully formed but still thin

BABY AT 8 WEEKS
Your baby's limbs are developing and the major organs are forming.

BABY AT 12 WEEKS
The facial features are apparent. Your baby has no layer of fat yet and the skin is translucent.

BABY AT 16 WEEKS
Your baby now resembles a tiny human being; nails are starting to grow on the fingers and toes.

BABY AT 24 WEEKS
Your baby is much larger now and very active. All the major organs are working, but the lungs and digestive system need to mature.

HOW IS THE AGE OF MY BABY CALCULATED?

The length of your pregnancy is calculated by an old convention that began when it was thought that conception occurred during your menstrual period. Although we now know that conception usually occurs just after ovulation, which occurs between nine and 18 days after the start of your last period, the old system is still used when your date of delivery is calculated. Therefore, the number of weeks you are pregnant and the age of the baby will always be worked out from the first day of your last period (see p. 17). Throughout this book, when discussing the age of your baby, we give the gestational (development) age as dated from the first day of your last menstrual period (LMP) – not the age of the embryo. These dates will therefore correspond with the dates given to you by your doctor or midwife and so avoid any confusion.

By this stage, most babies lie head down in the womb

There is not much space for movement in the womb

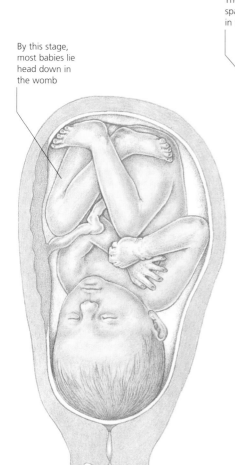

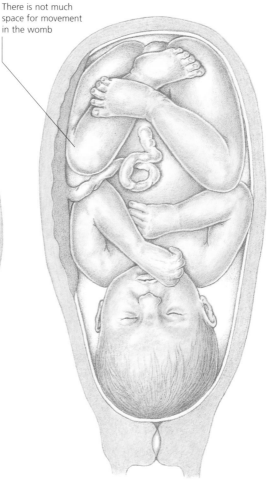

BABY AT 32 WEEKS
Your baby's head is now more in proportion to the body. Fat is accumulating under the skin. If born at this stage, your baby stands a very good chance of survival.

BABY AT 40 WEEKS
Now fully mature, much plumper and ready to emerge, your baby moves less and less as the surrounding fluid reduces and the womb is unable to expand further.

YOUR DEVELOPING BABY

Are there different stages of development?
Pregnancy is divided into three-month stages called trimesters. Your pregnancy has three trimesters of 12 or 13 weeks, each trimester being distinctly different as regards the development of you and your baby.

PREGNANCY TIMELINE
To help you find information about the precise developmental stage of both you and your baby, this chapter and the next one feature a timeline running along the bottom of each page. It is shaded to indicate which trimester you are reading about.

Pregnancy timeline

◻ First day of last period   ◼ Likely date of conception

WEEKS IN PREGNANCY

1	2	3	4	5	6	7	8	9	10	11	12	13	14	15	16	17	18	19	20	21	22	23	24	25	26	27	28	29	30	31	32	33	34	35	36	37	38	39	40

FIRST TRIMESTER	SECOND TRIMESTER	THIRD TRIMESTER

CONCEPTION

Q WHEN DOES CONCEPTION TAKE PLACE?

A You are most likely to conceive if sexual intercourse takes place when you are at your most fertile, that is, just after an egg has been released from a follicle in one of your ovaries; this usually happens around the middle of your menstrual cycle (see p. 12).

Q WHAT HAPPENS TO THE EGG WHEN IT IS RELEASED?

A Once the egg has been released from your ovaries, it is swept into the Fallopian tube and then slowly propelled down the tube by fine hairs (called cilia) that line the inside. These cilia act like a moving carpet, brushing the egg towards the womb.

HOW IS THE BABY'S SEX DETERMINED?

Chromosomes contain all the information needed to determine the genetic structure of the new baby. All human beings normally have two sex chromosomes – a combination of either an X and a Y (male), or an X and an X (female). The woman's egg always has an X chromosome, but sperm can have an X or a Y, so the sex of the baby will depend on whether it is an X or a Y sperm that penetrates the egg.

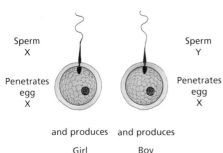

Sperm X — Penetrates egg X — and produces Girl XX

Sperm Y — Penetrates egg X — and produces Boy XY

X AND Y SPERM
The diagram above shows the penetration of the eggs by sperm containing either an X or a Y chromosome. The egg with an X sperm produces a girl, and with a Y sperm produces a boy.

Q HOW DOES FERTILIZATION TAKE PLACE?

A Once sperm are inside the vagina, they use their long tails to swim very rapidly through the cervix, along the inside of the womb, into the Fallopian tube, and then towards the released egg. The sperm are attracted to the egg by chemicals the egg produces. Several sperm may meet the egg at more or less the same time but, although many sperm cling to the egg's surface, only one sperm actually penetrates the egg's membrane; this is the point at which fertilization takes place.

Q WHERE DO THE SPERM AND EGG MEET?

A The sperm and egg normally meet in a Fallopian tube and this is where fertilization takes place. Occasionally, the sperm and egg meet and fertilize in other places, for example, at the ovary where the egg is released; this can cause an ectopic pregnancy (see p. 134), that is, a pregnancy that develops outside the womb. Fertilization usually has to take place within 36 hours of the egg being released from the ovary; after this time the egg is too old, and conception is unlikely to occur. Sperm can survive for up to three days in the womb.

Q WHAT HAPPENS AFTER FERTILIZATION?

A Once the sperm has penetrated the egg, the two cells fuse. The egg's outer membrane prevents any other sperm entering the egg. The fertilized egg then moves down the Fallopian tube into the womb and within a few days becomes a cluster (called a blastocyst) of about 60 cells. At around the time of your missed period, the blastocyst starts to glue itself to the inside wall of your womb; this is called implantation (see opposite). From here the cluster of cells will begin to develop into an embryo.

Q WHAT IF THE FERTILIZED EGG DOES NOT IMPLANT?

A Sometimes, in the complex events of fertilization and cell division, something goes wrong and a "non-viable" embryo (one that is unlikely to survive) is produced. When this occurs, the fertilized egg does not implant properly in the wall of the womb but continues on out of the womb. The only clue that this has happened may be a slightly late and heavy period.

WHAT HAPPENS AT CONCEPTION?

Life begins with the miracle of conception, when one sperm penetrates an egg's outer membrane and fuses with the egg. When the sperm and the egg (each of which has 23 chromosomes) fuse, the fertilized egg then has the full 46 chromosomes necessary to form a human being. Twins or multiple births occur when two or more eggs are fertilized at the same time. Identical twins occur when one fertilized egg divides into two and becomes two babies (see p. 66).

THE JOURNEY OF THE EGG

When the egg is first fertilized, as it journeys down the Fallopian tube to the womb, it is like a self-contained space capsule that survives on its own energy stores. At this stage, the egg is still microscopically small and can only just be seen by the human eye. After six days, just as the egg begins to exhaust its supply of energy, it attaches itself to the wall of the womb.

The beginning of life

The fertilized egg divides rapidly into two cells, then four, then eight, and so on. These early cells, when the fertilized egg (morula) is fewer than than 32 cells, have the ability to form any part of the baby's body and are known as "totipotential" cells.

Two cells

Four cells

Eight cells

Multi-celled

THE MOMENT OF CONCEPTION
Normally, only one sperm can break through the tough outer membrane of the egg; once the sperm enters the egg, the sperm loses its tail.

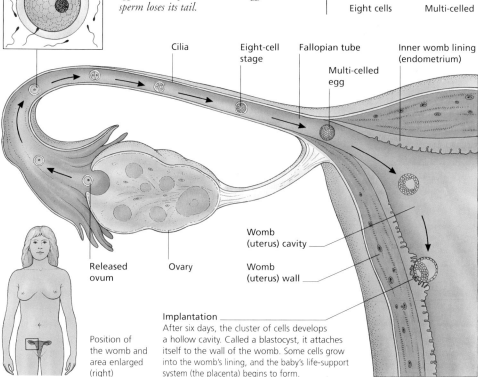

Cilia

Eight-cell stage

Fallopian tube

Multi-celled egg

Inner womb lining (endometrium)

Released ovum

Ovary

Womb (uterus) cavity

Womb (uterus) wall

Position of the womb and area enlarged (right)

Implantation
After six days, the cluster of cells develops a hollow cavity. Called a blastocyst, it attaches itself to the wall of the womb. Some cells grow into the womb's lining, and the baby's life-support system (the placenta) begins to form.

UP TO TWELVE WEEKS

YOUR BABY'S SIZE

Length (crown to rump)
6cm (2½in)
Weight 15g (½oz)

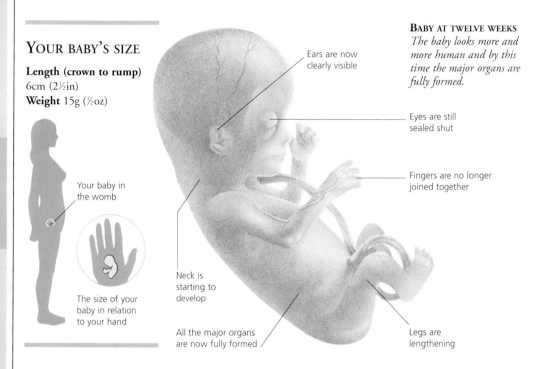

Your baby in the womb

The size of your baby in relation to your hand

Neck is starting to develop

All the major organs are now fully formed

Ears are now clearly visible

Eyes are still sealed shut

Fingers are no longer joined together

Legs are lengthening

BABY AT TWELVE WEEKS
The baby looks more and more human and by this time the major organs are fully formed.

HOW IS MY BABY GROWING?

What does my baby look like?
At twelve weeks the fetus looks like a tiny human being; it is about 6cm (2½in) long (crown to rump) and weighs about 15g (½oz). It has miniature arms and legs, with fingers, toes, and more defined facial features. The body is straighter and the first bone tissue appears. The head is still relatively large (about one third of the entire length of the body) but it is now supported by the suggestion of a neck.
■ **Face** The face is completely formed, with a chin, high forehead, and the small button nose of a young baby. The eyes are further developed and are at the front of the face, rather than the sides, but they are still widely spaced and shut tight by sealed eyelids. The ears are now higher on the side of the head.
■ **Arms and legs** These are now beginning to move.
■ **Skin and hair** The fetus' skin is red, translucent, and permeable to amniotic fluid.
■ **Feet and hands** The fingers and toes are by now more defined, and nails are starting to grow.

What is happening inside my baby's body?
By the end of the eleventh week of pregnancy, the main organs are completely formed but not all are fully functional.
■ **Heart** The heart is now completed and working, pumping blood to all parts of the body.
■ **Digestive system** The stomach has formed and is linked to the mouth and the intestines.
■ **Sexual organs** Ovaries or testes have formed inside the body, but although external sexual organs are developing, the baby's sex cannot yet be established visually on a scan.

The baby's life-support system
At around 12 weeks, the placenta has achieved its final shape and takes over from the yolk sac to become your baby's life-support system (see opposite). Much larger than the baby at this stage, the placenta is a thick disc-shaped organ attached to one area of the womb. After its initial rapid enlargement, the placenta's growth slows; by the time the baby is born, it weighs about one sixth of the baby's weight.

WEEKS IN PREGNANCY

1	2	3	4	5	6	7	8	9	10	11	12	13	14	15	16	17	18	19	20
				FIRST TRIMESTER														SECOND	

Q WHAT IS THE UMBILICAL CORD?

A The cord, which connects the placenta to the baby's navel, consists of three blood vessels that wind around each other. Two of the vessels are arteries taking blood from the baby to the placenta and one is a vein returning blood from the placenta to the baby. These vessels are surrounded by a thick protective substance called Wharton's jelly and encased in a further covering.

Q CAN KNOTS OCCUR IN MY BABY'S CORD?

A Yes, the cord can occasionally become knotted, but because the cord is very rubbery and slippery, the knot or knots are usually loose and cause no problem. Should the knot become tight during the birth, it can cause the baby distress by cutting off the supply of oxygen and nutrients. This is a rare occurrence but it can be linked to stillbirth before labour has started.

Q WHEN CAN I HEAR A HEARTBEAT?

A Your baby's heart can be heard by ten weeks with a device called a sonicaid. This uses Doppler ultrasound waves (see p. 34), which are high-frequency sound waves and quite harmless to your baby. At this early stage of development, your baby's heart rate is very fast, around 160 beats per minute. This rate slows as the baby grows.

Q WHEN DO THE BONES DEVELOP?

A The cartilage foundations are laid down in the body at about six weeks. Although the joints and bones are all formed in outline by 12 weeks, the process by which cartilage turns into hardened bone (ossification) takes far longer. Centres of hard bone are created while your baby is in the womb but at and after the birth the bones are still forming and will not be fully complete until adolescence.

YOUR DEVELOPING BABY

WHAT IS THE PLACENTA AND WHAT DOES IT DO?

The placenta is a marvellous piece of biological engineering. Attached to your womb wall and connected to your baby by the umbilical cord, it has several functions: it produces hormones that are vital to maintain the pregnancy; it acts as a filtering membrane, rather like the lungs, to breathe, digest, and excrete for your baby. Without ever mixing the maternal and fetal blood, it takes in oxygen and nutrients from your blood, and expels your baby's carbon dioxide and waste products.

HOW THE PLACENTA WORKS
Where the placenta adheres to the womb wall, it consists of very fine blood vessels containing the baby's blood. These are enveloped by pools of the mother's blood and this is where fluids, nutrients, and gases are exchanged.

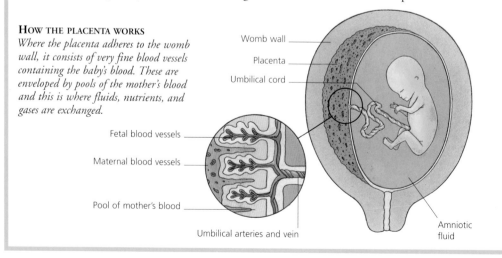

Womb wall
Placenta
Umbilical cord

Fetal blood vessels
Maternal blood vessels
Pool of mother's blood
Umbilical arteries and vein

Amniotic fluid

WEEKS IN PREGNANCY

21	22	23	24	25	26	27	28	29	30	31	32	33	34	35	36	37	38	39	40

TRIMESTER · THIRD TRIMESTER

53

UP TO SIXTEEN WEEKS

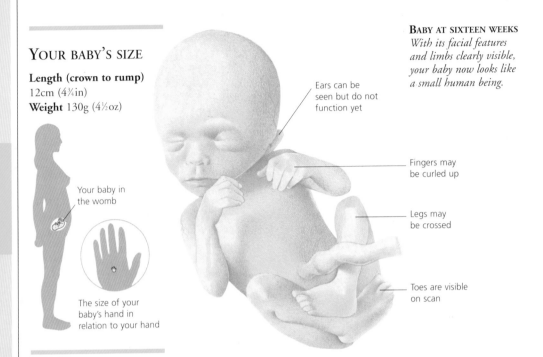

BABY AT SIXTEEN WEEKS
With its facial features and limbs clearly visible, your baby now looks like a small human being.

YOUR BABY'S SIZE

Length (crown to rump)
12cm (4¾in)
Weight 130g (4½oz)

Your baby in the womb

The size of your baby's hand in relation to your hand

Ears can be seen but do not function yet

Fingers may be curled up

Legs may be crossed

Toes are visible on scan

HOW IS MY BABY GROWING?

What does my baby look like?
By 16 weeks your baby is about 12cm (4¾in) long (crown to rump), and weighs about 130g (4½oz). Although the baby is still very small, all the limbs and features are formed, and are more in proportion. Because there is no layer of fat, the baby will look thin; the skin is so fine and translucent that underlying blood vessels can be clearly seen. The baby is also very active and can make a fist, suck a thumb, swallow fluid, and excrete into the amniotic fluid.
■ **Head** The facial bones have formed, so a scan at this stage may reveal more delicate features, such as the nose or mouth. Because the facial muscles have developed, the baby can make – but not control – expressions. The eyes are becoming sensitive to changes in light, even though they are still shut tight. Very fine eyebrows and eyelashes have started to grow; tastebuds appear on the tongue. By 16 weeks, the small bones in the ear harden and your baby hears some first sounds.

■ **Arms and legs** The legs have now caught up with arm development, and become longer than the arms. Tiny fingernails are appearing at the end of delicate fingers, but the toenails begin to grow later.

What is happening inside my baby's body?
The baby's range of movements greatly increases due to the development of the nervous system.
■ **Nervous system** A layer of fat (myelin) is beginning to coat the nerves that link muscles to the brain. This is important because once the connections are complete, messages can be passed to and from the brain, allowing co-ordinated movement.

The baby's life-support system
Inside the sac of membranes, your baby is surrounded by protective amniotic fluid, which means that he or she can move about freely and develop muscle tone. Your baby may be head down one minute and feet down the next but you are unlikely to feel any of the movements yet because the fluid cushions you from these tiny sensations.

WEEKS IN PREGNANCY

1	2	3	4	5	6	7	8	9	10	11	12	13	14	15	16	17	18	19	20

FIRST TRIMESTER	SECOND

Q WHY IS MY BABY SURROUNDED BY FLUID?

A The amniotic fluid protects your baby from knocks, and keeps the temperature in your womb steady. Until 14 weeks the amniotic fluid is absorbed through the baby's delicate skin. After this time, as the kidneys start to work, the baby swallows and excretes the fluid back into the amniotic cavity. Although the amount of fluid around your baby is relatively stable, it is constantly absorbed and replaced and never becomes stale. Until around the thirty-fourth week there is enough to allow your baby to move around and develop the muscles.

Q WHY DOESN'T A BABY DROWN IN THE SURROUNDING FLUID?

A Your baby cannot actually breathe yet and instead obtains all its oxygen from the blood in the placenta. Imagine the baby as a diver immersed in water, and using the placenta as an oxygen tank; the only difference between your baby and a diver is that the baby's oxygen is passed directly into the circulatory system via the placenta, by-passing the lungs.

Q WHAT CAN MY BABY DO AT THIS STAGE?

A All the connections between your baby's brain, nervous system, and muscles are established by now, allowing for a far more intricate range of movements. He or she will be able to flex and extend fingers, arms, and legs. If you have a scan, you may even be able to see your baby sucking his or her thumb, or appearing to grasp the umbilical cord. The baby's bladder is filling and emptying with amniotic fluid as a rehearsal for its eventual role.

Q CAN I FEEL MY BABY'S MOVEMENTS THIS EARLY ON?

A It is rare to feel any movement as early as this because although your baby can move in a reasonably co-ordinated way from about 13 weeks, the surrounding amniotic fluid cushions these small movements. Some women say that they can feel very light sensations like "butterflies" in their lower abdomen at around 16 weeks, but this is unusual. As your baby grows, you will be able to feel the movements become more and more definite.

DISCUSSION POINT

WHAT AFFECTS MY BABY'S SIZE?

Family and medical reasons

Your baby's size is dependent on many different factors, although genetics usually determine the size of a baby, which is related to the size of the mother. Therefore, if you are small in stature, your baby is also likely to be small, and if you are tall, you are likely to have a larger baby. You will probably have a small baby if you yourself are small but your partner is very tall. If you have already had a baby, subsequent babies will tend to be heavier than the earlier one and boys tend to weigh more than girls at delivery. However, the birthweight does not necessarily relate to the eventual size of the adult. Medical conditions can also have a major effect on your baby's size; pre-eclampsia, for example (see p. 127), can result in a small baby, and diabetes can cause a baby to be large (see p. 125).

Other factors

Your lifestyle and environment can also affect the size of your baby. What and how you eat is important for your baby's welfare. If you eat a balanced diet, your baby should receive all the necessary nutrients to be able to grow to the optimum size. However, if you are malnourished, you can have a low birthweight baby and there may be problems with the baby's health. Regular heavy smoking can cause small babies because smoking reduces the amount of oxygen and nutrients reaching the baby. For each cigarette smoked per day, the baby's weight will be reduced on average by 13g (½oz). Your ethnic origin can also influence the size of your baby; for example, for genetic and dietary reasons, women from Asia tend to have smaller babies than those of Scandinavian and American origin.

21	22	23	24	25	26	27	28	29	30	31	32	33	34	35	36	37	38	39	40

TRIMESTER | THIRD TRIMESTER

UP TO TWENTY WEEKS

YOUR DEVELOPING BABY

YOUR BABY'S SIZE

Length (crown to rump)
16cm (6⅓in)
Weight 340g (12 oz)

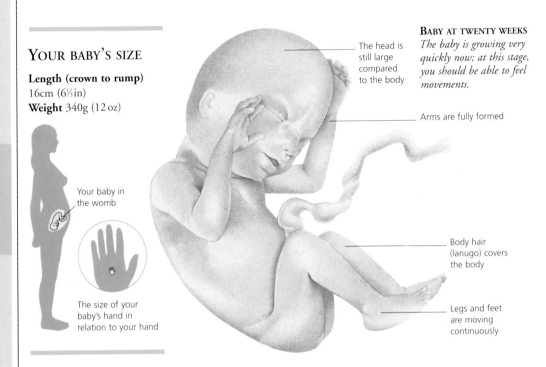

Your baby in the womb

The size of your baby's hand in relation to your hand

The head is still large compared to the body

BABY AT TWENTY WEEKS
The baby is growing very quickly now; at this stage, you should be able to feel movements.

Arms are fully formed

Body hair (lanugo) covers the body

Legs and feet are moving continuously

HOW IS MY BABY GROWING?

What does my baby look like?
By 20 weeks your baby will be about 16cm (6⅓in) long (crown to rump), and weigh approximately 340g (12oz). The growth rate, which has so far been very fast, now slows down to allow the lungs, digestive system, and immune system more time to mature. Your baby can now hear acutely and loud bangs will make him or her jump. You should feel these movements very clearly.
■ **Head and face** The eyes are still shut but eye movements have developed enabling your baby's eyes to move slowly from side to side. The taste buds are very well developed and the first teeth have now formed within the gums.
■ **Body** Your baby is not quite as thin as last month because it has developed a layer of fat. Some of this is brownish-coloured (brown fat) and appears around the nape of the neck, the kidneys, and behind the breastbone. Layers of ordinary (white) fat are also building up on the rest of the body.

■ **Skin and hair** The skin is covered by fine downy hair known as lanugo, and a protective waxy coating of thick white cream known as the vernix (see p. 63).

What is happening inside my baby's body?
Movements are far more co-ordinated and the baby's own reproductive organs are developing rapidly.
■ **Movements** Your baby will be much more active and have far greater control because the muscles and nervous system are more developed. Most of the major organs are now functioning.
■ **Sexual organs** These are now well developed and are usually visible on a scan. In a girl, the ovaries will now hold all her eggs (about seven million at this stage) and the nipples and mammary glands appear.

Your baby's life-support system
From now on, the fully developed placenta will provide all your baby's needs until birth; in addition to providing oxygen, nutrients, and protective antibodies, it disposes of waste products. Although the placenta continues to grow, it is now smaller than the baby.

WEEKS IN PREGNANCY

1	2	3	4	5	6	7	8	9	10	11	12	13	14	15	16	17	18	19	20
			FIRST TRIMESTER															SECOND	

Q WHEN WILL I BE ABLE TO FEEL MY BABY MOVING?

A You may not be able to feel your baby moving properly before 22 weeks, although you may sometimes detect occasional "flutterings" from about 16 weeks onwards. If you have had a baby before, you may be more aware of these light movements. However, you will not notice any regular movements until about 24 weeks, so you should try not to worry about how much your baby is moving at this stage.

Q WHEN DOES MY BABY START TO GROW ANY HAIR?

A The first hairs appear around the baby's eyebrows and upper lip from about 14 weeks onwards. By around 20 weeks, the baby is covered all over by fine hair. This hair, called lanugo, is shed at birth. Both lanugo and the baby's head hair (which may be scarce or plentiful at birth) are entirely replaced by new, coarser hair growing out of new hair follicles within the first three months.

Q WHEN WILL I KNOW WHETHER MY BABY IS NORMAL OR NOT?

A Most babies are born perfectly normal and healthy. An ultrasound scan at 18 to 20 weeks, is usually detailed enough to allow many major abnormalities to be detected; this scan will also allow your doctor to check the major organs such as the brain and heart. If there is any question of a chromosomal or genetic problem (see p. 35), further tests are usually done during this trimester. If all these tests are clear, it is very likely that your baby is normal. However, it is important to understand that no test can guarantee a problem-free baby, as some minor defects cannot be detected before birth (see p. 132).

QUESTIONS TO ASK

Is my baby the right size for my dates?

Is my baby moving enough?

Where is the placenta situated?

Are my baby's major organs developing well?

Is there enough amniotic fluid around my baby?

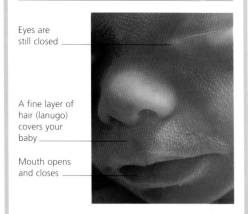

WHAT YOU CAN SEE

Eyes are still closed

A fine layer of hair (lanugo) covers your baby

Mouth opens and closes

AT TWENTY WEEKS
If you were to see a photograph or have a scan of your baby at around 18 to 20 weeks, you would see that the facial features are very clear. It may even be possible to see the baby's tongue poking out through parted lips.

Q CAN MY BABY FEEL COLD IN THE WOMB?

A This is unlikely because your baby is protected by your body, and also bathed in warm amniotic fluid so that there is a consistent, temperature-controlled environment.

Q IS MY BABY AWARE OF ANYTHING OUTSIDE THE WOMB?

A Babies can hear, and do respond, to acoustic (sound) stimulation from the end of the first trimester; they respond by moving, or their heartbeats can change. Some mothers report that their babies change the pattern of their movements in response to different kinds of music.

Q CAN MY BABY SEE ANYTHING?

A Until about 22 weeks, your baby's eyelids are shut. After this time your baby can't see much, partly because it is very dark, and also because babies have a limited visual range until a few weeks after birth. However, it is thought that babies are aware of sunlight and darkness in the womb.

WEEKS IN PREGNANCY

21	22	23	24	25	26	27	28	29	30	31	32	33	34	35	36	37	38	39	40

TRIMESTER | THIRD TRIMESTER

UP TO TWENTY-FOUR WEEKS

YOUR BABY'S SIZE

Length (crown to rump)
21cm (8in)
Weight 630g (1lb 6 oz)

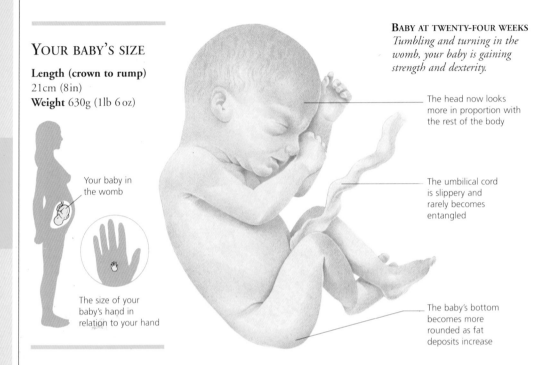

Your baby in
the womb

The size of your
baby's hand in
relation to your hand

BABY AT TWENTY-FOUR WEEKS
*Tumbling and turning in the
womb, your baby is gaining
strength and dexterity.*

The head now looks
more in proportion with
the rest of the body

The umbilical cord
is slippery and
rarely becomes
entangled

The baby's bottom
becomes more
rounded as fat
deposits increase

HOW IS MY BABY GROWING?

What does my baby look like?
By 24 weeks, your baby has become less delicate and
has probably gained about 500g (1lb) in weight in the
last month; it is now about 21cm (8in) long (crown
to rump) and weighs about 630g (1lb 6oz).
■ **Skin** Still fine, but no longer translucent, the baby's
skin is now reddish in colour and, because layers of
fat have yet to form, rather wrinkly.
■ **Eyes** At 22 to 24 weeks, your baby's eyes open.

What is happening inside my baby's body?
Surrounded by about 500ml (18fl oz) of amniotic fluid
your baby can move around inside your womb with
great mobility. He or she can kick, suck a thumb, open
and close the mouth, and will respond to movement
or loud noises. The heart rate has dropped to about
140–150 beats per minute, and it is now possible to
get a print-out of your baby's heart rate on a CTG
(cardiotocograph) machine. All the major organs
(except the lungs) are now functioning.

■ **Brain and nervous system** If the brainwaves of
your 24 week-old baby are viewed on a special
monitoring machine called an EEG (electro-
encephalogram), they would resemble those of a
newborn infant. The cells that control conscious
thought are developing, and your baby becomes much
more sensitive to sound and movement and, by this
stage, is also thought to have developed a cycle of
sleeping and waking.
■ **Lungs** The lungs, which are still full of amniotic
fluid, are the least mature organs and still have several
weeks before all the small air exchange sacs (alveoli)
are completely formed.
■ **Digestive system** Your baby is constantly
swallowing and excreting amniotic fluid.

The baby's life-support system
The walls of the tiny blood vessels (villi) of the
placental tissue become thinner and more permeable
as the pregnancy progresses, so that the amount of
nutrients passed to the baby increases and greater
quantities of waste are eliminated.

WEEKS IN PREGNANCY

1	2	3	4	5	6	7	8	9	10	11	12	13	14	15	16	17	18	19	20
FIRST TRIMESTER												SECOND							

Q WHAT IS THE EARLIEST AGE AT WHICH BABIES CAN SURVIVE IF BORN EARLY?

A The legal definition of viability (the age at which a baby can survive outside the womb) is 24 weeks and after. A baby born before this time is unlikely to survive and the mother will be considered to have had a miscarriage. At 24 weeks, there is a possibility of damage to the baby's internal organs during labour and the baby may be physically or mentally disabled. If you give birth after 24 weeks, you are considered to have had a premature labour and your baby may be put in a special care unit, possibly in an incubator (see p. 214). After 28 weeks, the risks decrease and the prospects for the baby's survival are very good (over 90 per cent).

Q CAN MY BABY DEVELOP IMMUNITY TO INFECTIONS WHILE IN THE WOMB?

A Your body provides certain antibodies that cross the placenta and provide your baby with immunity during the pregnancy and for several months after delivery (breastfeeding augments this protection). Your baby can produce antibodies while in the womb, but this usually only happens if you contract an infection to which you and your baby have no immunity.

Q IS IT QUIET IN THE WOMB?

A On the contrary, evidence suggests that the womb is very noisy. With the sound of your blood whooshing through your arteries and through the placenta, the continuous humming of blood along major veins, as well as the gurgling of your bowels, it is probably comparable to being underwater in a swimming pool. Your baby can also hear voices, and learns to identify your voice and that of your partner.

Q WHY IS MY BUMP BIGGER/SMALLER THAN THOSE OF OTHER WOMEN?

A Some women have a large bulge at 24 weeks, others seem to hide the pregnancy completely until 30 weeks or later! It all depends on your body shape and how thin or overweight you are, the strength of your abdominal wall muscles, and the size of your baby or babies. If your doctor or midwife confirms that your baby is growing normally, don't worry about comparisons with other bumps – it really does not matter.

WHAT YOU CAN SEE

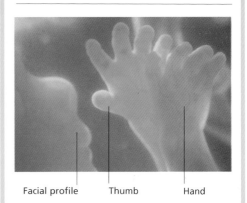

Facial profile   Thumb   Hand

AT TWENTY-ONE WEEKS
A photograph taken of your baby in the womb at this time (like the one above) would show that your baby's fingers are now fully formed and can grasp. This baby seems to be holding on to the umbilical cord.

Q WILL MY BABY GROW BIGGER AND HEALTHIER IF I EAT MORE?

A Unless you have been severely malnourished, and you suddenly start eating a tremendous amount of food, the answer is no. As long as your diet is providing the basic nutrients, your baby will continue to grow at a steady rate regardless of what you actually eat (see p. 100). However, it is important not to eat too much during your pregnancy; if you become seriously overweight, you increase the risk of developing a condition called gestational diabetes (see p. 125). Also, if your baby has to be delivered by a Caesarean section, being very overweight can make the operation more complicated.

Q WHY ARE SOME BABIES MORE ACTIVE IN THE WOMB THAN OTHERS?

A This is a difficult question to answer. Some babies do seem to move more than others, but the reason for this is not clear. However, it is also true that some women simply feel their babies moving more, whereas other women do not feel their babies moving even when they have done a complete somersault in the womb.

WEEKS IN PREGNANCY

21	22	23	24	25	26	27	28	29	30	31	32	33	34	35	36	37	38	39	40

TRIMESTER	THIRD TRIMESTER

Up to Twenty-nine weeks

Your baby's size

Length (crown to rump)
26 cm (10 in)
Weight 1.1kg (2lb 7oz)

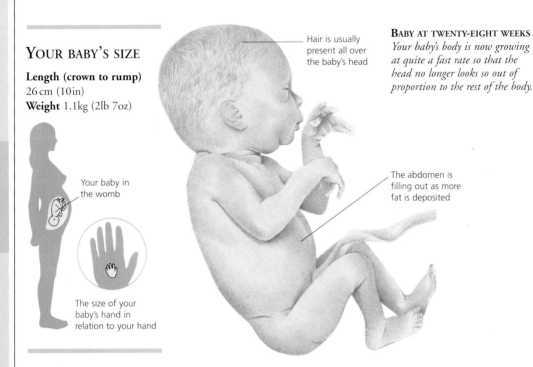

Your baby in
the womb

The size of your
baby's hand in
relation to your hand

Hair is usually
present all over
the baby's head

The abdomen is
filling out as more
fat is deposited

BABY AT TWENTY-EIGHT WEEKS
*Your baby's body is now growing
at quite a fast rate so that the
head no longer looks so out of
proportion to the rest of the body.*

How is my baby growing?

What does my baby look like?
By 29 weeks your baby is about 26cm (10in) long
(crown to rump) and weighs about 1.1kg (2lb 7oz);
a greasy substance called vernix covers and
insulates the baby's skin (see p. 63). If born now,
your baby should be physically developed enough
to survive, but would require special care.

What is happening inside my baby's body?
Your baby moves around regularly in the womb.
■ **Brain** This grows much larger, and a fatty
protective sheath covers the nerve fibres; this
important development allows brain impulses
to travel faster, enhancing the ability to learn.
■ **Movements** Your baby is now more cramped in
the womb due to the increase in length and weight.
However, your baby can still change position; less
cushioning fluid means that you will begin to feel
these movements more and they may even be
visible from the outside.

■ **Lungs** At 29 weeks, the lungs have developed most
of their smaller airways and tiny air sacs (alveoli).
Equally important is the development of a substance
called surfactant, which is produced by cells in the
lungs. Surfactant assists with breathing by reducing
the surface tension of the lining of the lungs; this
prevents the airways in the lungs from collapsing
when breath is exhaled. A premature baby may have
problems with breathing because this substance has
not been produced. In a premature birth, either a
steroid injection is given to the mother to stimulate
the baby's lungs to produce surfactant, or the baby
is given artificial surfactant at birth.

The baby's life-support system
At this stage the placenta grows at a slower rate than
your baby. It receives about 400ml (14fl oz) of blood
from your circulation every minute and exchanges
nutrients, gases, and waste products. The placenta
is quite selective in what it allows to pass from the
mother to the baby's blood, stopping some harmful
substances, such as certain drugs, from crossing over.

WEEKS IN PREGNANCY

1	2	3	4	5	6	7	8	9	10	11	12	13	14	15	16	17	18	19	20
				FIRST TRIMESTER															SECOND

Q SHOULD MY BABY STILL BE MOVING?

A Yes, at 29 weeks your baby should feel very active. It is only after 36 weeks that your baby will quieten down because, by this stage, there will be less space and therefore less amniotic fluid to move around in. You may see your baby move if your bump heaves and bulges, and you can often feel him or her moving under your hand.

Q CAN MY BABY DAMAGE ME BY KICKING AND MOVING?

A Although vigorous movement is common after about 28 weeks, your baby will not injure you because the amniotic fluid will absorb any kicks, and the thick muscular wall of the womb will protect your stomach, liver, and bowels.

Q I SOMETIMES FEEL A SHARP PAIN UNDER MY RIBS. SHOULD I BE CONCERNED?

A If your baby is head down (cephalic) and he or she kicks, it can sometimes hurt you just below the ribs. Occasionally, pain beneath your ribs can be caused by your baby's head bobbing around in the breech position (see p. 63). This isn't dangerous but it can be uncomfortable. Sometimes a sharp pain under the ribs is the only sign that your baby is breech.

Q IF MY BABY IS HEAD DOWN AT THIS STAGE, IS IT GOING TO STAY THAT WAY?

A No, not necessarily. At this stage, the baby is still able to move around and will continue to move until about 35 to 36 weeks; after this time, your baby is too big to move easily and usually settles into one position ready for labour.

Q WHY DO BABIES GET HICCUPS?

A Babies do have occasional short, jerky "hiccups" which you can sometimes feel. They are probably caused by the baby moving the chest in an attempt to practise breathing. These movements can be seen on an ultrasound scan, and are thought to allow the baby's lungs to expand and develop properly. However, the baby doesn't need to breathe in the proper sense until born because oxygen is carried through the placenta straight into the baby's blood system via the umbilical cord.

WHAT A SCAN SHOWS

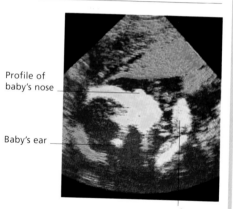

Profile of baby's nose

Baby's ear

Arm

AT TWENTY-FOUR WEEKS
This ultrasound scan shows the profile of a baby around six months. By this stage, all facial features are formed, so that he or she will look much the same now as at birth, only smaller. The eyes are still shut, but will open in the next few weeks.

Q DO BOYS AND GIRLS WEIGH THE SAME?

A Boy babies during the third trimester of pregnancy usually weigh slightly more than girls at the same number of weeks.

Q WHAT DOES IT MEAN IF MY BABY IS SAID TO BE SMALL FOR ITS DATES?

A This means that your baby is smaller than is typical for its number of weeks. The most common reason for this is genetic: your baby was never meant to be big in the first place. This is especially true if you and/or your partner are short or underweight. Another possible cause is that the placenta isn't functioning properly, therefore the baby is not getting enough nutrients and oxygen. This is called "placental insufficiency" and is sometimes, but not always, linked to the development of pre-eclampsia (see p. 127). A possible but less likely reason is that your dates are wrong and you are, in fact, less far advanced in pregnancy than everyone thinks. Rarely, an infection, chromosomal, or genetic problem can hinder a baby's growth (see p. 52).

YOUR DEVELOPING BABY

21	22	23	24	25	26	27	28	29	30	31	32	33	34	35	36	37	38	39	40

WEEKS IN PREGNANCY

TRIMESTER · THIRD TRIMESTER

TWINS AND MULTIPLE BIRTHS

Q AM I MORE LIKELY TO HAVE TWINS IF THERE ARE TWINS IN MY FAMILY?

A Yes, you are. Non-identical twins are more likely if a close relative has had twins or triplets, or if you are a non-identical twin. However, the incidence of identical twins is more random and not always linked to your family history.

Q HOW COMMON ARE TWINS?

A Twins are more common in women who conceive after the age of 35, or have had fertility treatments, such as IVF and GIFT (see p. 15); over half of triplets result from assisted conception techniques. Although the reason for this is not clear, multiple pregnancies are also more common in certain parts of the world such as Nigeria, where 45 per 1,000 births are twins. In Europe the rate is about 10 per 1,000.

Q WHEN WILL MY DOCTOR CONFIRM THAT I'M EXPECTING TWINS?

A It is possible to see twins on an ultrasound scan at about eight weeks. However, because there is a higher risk of miscarriage (of one or both babies), a diagnosis of "viable" twins is rarely made until the beginning of the second trimester, at 12 to 14 weeks.

Q WHAT ARE THE RISKS INVOLVED IN HAVING TWINS?

A If you are expecting twins, you are considered to be a high-risk pregnancy. Extra demands are placed on the mother and the placental system on which the babies rely. In turn this can slow the growth of one or both the babies, and cause high blood pressure in the mother. There is also a strong chance of premature birth. These risks are further compounded with triplets or even higher multiple pregnancies (see p. 130).

HOW DO TWINS DEVELOP?

Twins develop at an early stage when, or just after, the egg and sperm meet. Twins are either non-identical (more common, accounting for about 80 per cent of twins) or identical (less frequent, about 20 per cent). The twins below are in a vertex (head down) position, but they can also occupy other positions in the womb (see p. 185).

IDENTICAL TWINS

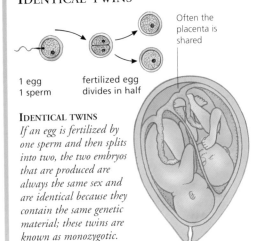

1 egg
1 sperm

fertilized egg
divides in half

Often the placenta is shared

IDENTICAL TWINS
If an egg is fertilized by one sperm and then splits into two, the two embryos that are produced are always the same sex and are identical because they contain the same genetic material; these twins are known as monozygotic.

FRATERNAL TWINS

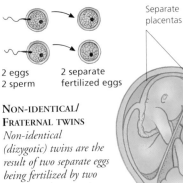

2 eggs
2 sperm

2 separate
fertilized eggs

Separate placentas

**NON-IDENTICAL/
FRATERNAL TWINS**
Non-identical (dizygotic) twins are the result of two separate eggs being fertilized by two sperms at the same time, so that two embryos implant and develop. The twins may look different and be different sexes.

Q IS A MULTIPLE PREGNANCY ALWAYS HIGH-RISK?

A Yes, you will be under the very close eye of an obstetrician, and have regular scans and clinic visits. It also means that a home birth will not be recommended.

Q WILL TWO BABIES BE ABLE TO DEVELOP PROPERLY IN MY WOMB?

A Your womb is amazingly stretchy and it is quite possible for two, and sometimes three (or more) babies to grow and develop quite normally; there is usually no problem in their development as long as each is surrounded by a separate protective sac of amniotic fluid (see below). It is, however, much more likely that you will go into labour before 40 weeks because the amount of space in your womb is limited.

Q CAN THE TWINS KNOCK INTO OR HURT EACH OTHER IN THE WOMB?

A Your twins can bump into each other in your womb, because they will be quite active. During a scan they may even seem to be playing with each other. However, they cannot hurt each other because they each have their own sac and fluid.

Q DOES IT MATTER IF MY TWINS ARE IDENTICAL OR NOT?

A Yes, it is important because if they are identical and share the same placenta and amniotic sac, they may encounter more problems with their development and delivery than non-identical twins (see p. 130). For this reason, if you are pregnant with identical twins, you will be closely monitored and you can expect frequent scans.

Q WHY DID MY EARLY SCAN SHOW TWINS, AND NOW ONLY ONE BABY SHOWS?

A Twin pregnancies may develop more often than we think, but at an early stage one twin dies or doesn't develop. As the surviving twin grows, the non-viable twin is "reabsorbed" and disappears with almost no trace. In the first trimester this shouldn't cause problems, but if a twin dies later in pregnancy, difficulties may occur (see p. 130).

Q DO TWINS AND TRIPLETS DEVELOP AT THE SAME RATE AS SINGLE BABIES?

A Yes, they develop in exactly the same way, at the same rate except that they may not grow quite as large as single babies, even taking into account the fact that they are usually born earlier.

Q DO TWINS SHARE THE SAME SAC OF AMNIOTIC FLUID?

A Non-identical twins, being the result of two eggs fertilized by two separate sperm which develop independently of each other, have separate umbilical cords, placentas, and amniotic sacs. Although identical twins, which are the result of one egg fertilized by a single sperm that has divided to form two or more embryos, share a placenta, they always have their own cord and usually their own sac.

Q I'M TOLD THAT MY TWINS ARE GROWING AT DIFFERENT RATES, WHY IS THIS?

A Twins may be different sizes to start off with, and can also grow at different rates. This is why if you have twins, you are offered frequent scans. It isn't usually a problem if both babies start off at different sizes but grow at normal rates; however, it may become a problem if they were both the same size initially, and one suddenly starts to grow much slower than the other (see below).

Q WHAT HAPPENS IF ONE TWIN IS GROWING MORE SLOWLY?

A If there is "discrepant growth", you will be scanned frequently and, depending on the well-being of the smaller, less healthy twin, the twins may be delivered early. In identical twins, a big difference in size may suggest a rare condition called "twin-to-twin transfusion syndrome", caused by an abnormal blood vessel connection (see p. 131).

Q IS IT TRUE THAT I WILL BE ABLE TO FEEL MY TWINS MOVING SEPARATELY?

A Because of each baby's own specific patterns of movement and relative position in the womb, many mothers can identify which baby is moving at a particular time. Twins do move separately; often one can be fast asleep or not moving much while the other is bouncing around.

QUESTIONS TO ASK

Are my babies growing at the same rate?

Are my twins identical or non-identical?

Is there a normal amount of amniotic fluid around each twin?

Are they the same sex or different sexes?

Have I got one or two placentas?

COMMON COMPLAINTS

Q MY BUMP IS NOW HUGE AND I AM VERY UNCOMFORTABLE – WHAT CAN I DO?

A There is little you can do about the discomfort in the final phase of your pregnancy because your baby is now very large and takes up a lot of space in your abdomen. Lying on your back may no longer be possible or advisable because the weight of your womb presses on the main blood vessel. This causes your blood pressure to drop, which in turn can make you feel faint. By this stage of pregnancy, your baby is probably also pushing out your ribs, causing them to ache. There are positions you can adopt to ease some of the pressure (see p. 113). It may also help to know that if your baby engages, a few of these discomforts should ease.

HOW CAN I RELIEVE CRAMP?

Cramp is the excruciating pain of muscles in spasm. The causes of cramp are uncertain but may be linked to low calcium levels. Cramp often occurs in bed at night, and particularly if you point your toes.

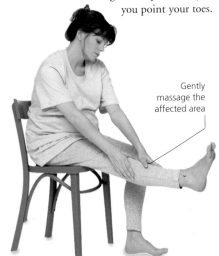

Gently massage the affected area

WHAT TO DO
To help relax the muscle that is in spasm, try extending the leg and then bringing the toes towards your body. Having a glass of milk (which contains calcium) can ease leg cramps.

Q IS IT NORMAL TO BE SHORT OF BREATH ALL THE TIME?

A It is normal to feel that you are not breathing deeply enough. Also, as your womb continues to expand into your abdomen, it presses against your diaphragm and your lungs, and this also makes it more difficult for you to take deep breaths. The increase in the hormone progesterone may also speed up your breathing (see p. 73).

Q WHY ARE THE PALMS OF MY HANDS RED AND BURNING?

A You have what is called palmar erythema; this occurs because of the increased blood flow through the skin tissues. It is not serious, but is just a result of the changes in your blood vessels.

Q I SEEM TO BE CONSTANTLY ITCHING ALL OVER – IS THERE SOMETHING WRONG?

A As your belly expands, your skin stretches to accommodate the growing baby; this stretching can make the skin itchy. Creams, calamine lotion, and bath oils can moisturize the skin, helping to reduce this itching. Rarely, severe generalized itching, especially late in pregnancy, needs to be seen by your doctor because it could indicate a liver disease (see p. 126).

Q I'VE DEVELOPED PILES, CAN I DO ANYTHING TO RELIEVE THEM?

A Piles (haemorrhoids) are varicose veins in the back passage that swell when the weight of the baby puts pressure on the main veins in the pelvis; this pressure in turn reduces the return of blood from the pelvic organs to the heart. Piles can be painful and delivery of your baby is really the only cure. Avoid constipation as this will add to your discomfort. Your doctor can prescribe soothing ointments for piles; if they ache, sit for ten minutes on an ice pack or bag of frozen peas wrapped in a towel. Pelvic floor exercises may help to reduce piles (see p. 107).

Q MY HEARTBEAT FEELS UNEVEN SOMETIMES – IS THIS UNUSUAL?

A "Missed" beats are also called palpitations, and normally they are nothing to worry about. However, if your heart starts missing beats very frequently, or you feel breathless or have chest pain with these palpitations, you should see your doctor.

WEEKS IN PREGNANCY

1	2	3	4	5	6	7	8	9	10	11	12	13	14	15	16	17	18	19	2
FIRST TRIMESTER																		SECON	

WHY DO MY BACK AND HIPS ACHE?

Throughout your pregnancy, hormones relax the ligaments and joints, particularly those in the pelvis, causing the ligaments to soften and stretch to allow the baby an easier passage in labour. Added to which, the weight of your growing baby can weaken your stomach muscles and put pressure on your lower back. As your centre of gravity changes, you may also tend to lean backwards, which can result in further strain. If your back pain is constant or severe, consult your doctor: it may be necessary to see a physiotherapist or an osteopath for help with pain relief.

TYPES OF BACK AND JOINT ACHE

Sacroiliac joint
Steady pain in middle/low back
Where your pelvis meets the lower spine (the sacrum), there are joints on either side called sacroiliac joints. In pregnancy, these can become unstable, which can be very painful, especially when walking, standing or bending.

Treatment Wear low-heeled shoes and ensure correct posture (see p. 110). If in severe pain, see your doctor, a physiotherapist or an osteopath.

Coccyx
Pain in the lower spine
The coccyx can become slightly displaced from the sacrum, causing excruciating pain especially when sitting. This type of pain usually results from previous injury.

Treatment You can take a pain-relieving drug, such as paracetamol. After pregnancy, an osteopath may be able to help.

Pubic joint
Pain in the front of the pelvis
The pelvis is made up of fused bones which form a ring-like structure; at the front, where the bones meet, is the symphysis pubis. If the ligaments around this joint loosen in late pregnancy, the pubic bones rub against each other, causing severe pain when you walk. Rarely, these bones separate: this is called diastasis of the symphysis pubis.

Treatment This usually requires consultation with a doctor or physiotherapist. You may have to wear a special support belt to relieve the pressure, or you may need further treatment.

Sciatic nerves
Sharp/constant/intermittent pain in the back, buttocks, and legs
As your baby's head moves down into your pelvis, it often presses directly on the pelvic bones, which may affect the sciatic nerves in your lower back and legs. This can cause severe back and leg pain, or your legs may feel numb. This is called sciatic nerve pain (see p. 120).

Treatment The best way of dealing with this is to spend some time lying down on a firm mattress. Your baby's head may move and relieve the pressure on the nerves; the pelvic tilt exercise may also help (see p. 108).

YOUR CHANGING BODY

1	22	23	24	25	26	27	28	29	30	31	32	33	34	35	36	37	38	39	40

TRIMESTER | THIRD TRIMESTER

FAMILY CHANGES

Q HOW SHOULD I PREPARE MY CHILD FOR THE NEW BABY'S ARRIVAL?

A First, tell your child that a new baby is on the way and explain what this will mean; then prepare for changes in your child's routine. You need to handle these issues positively but with great care and sensitivity. What you say and how you say it will obviously depend on the age of your child (see opposite).

Q WHY IS IT IMPORTANT TO PREPARE MY CHILD FOR THE NEW BABY'S ARRIVAL?

A After the birth of your baby, your child will undergo a major change in his or her life. After all, your first child has been an only child for all of his life and has enjoyed not only all your attention but also that of close family and friends. Whatever the age of your child, he or she has been your "baby" for some time and is now expected to relinquish that role to become a big brother or sister. This can seem a very poor deal.

Q HOW IS MY CHILD LIKELY TO REACT?

A The chances are that you will be faced with mixed emotions, ranging from excitement at having a new playmate, to worry that the new baby will be your favourite child. Your child may appear to be unaffected by the news but then go through a bout of naughtiness, or be unable to comprehend that a new baby is on its way and not react until after the birth. Or you may hear your child proudly tell friends that he or she is going to have a sister or brother. Whatever the reaction, your child will need reassurance and understanding from you.

Q HOW DO I CHANGE MY CHILD'S ROUTINE TO MANAGE THE NEW BABY?

A If you are planning any major changes in your child's routine, try to do this months before your baby is born. For instance, if you want your child to move from a cot to a bed, to start at nursery, or to go to bed earlier every night, try to establish these new routines months ahead of the birth or these upsets will become inextricably linked with the baby's arrival. Alternatively, you could leave any changes in your child's routine until a few months after the birth.

Q I HAVE A TEENAGE CHILD – WILL A NEW BABY CAUSE PROBLEMS?

A Some teenagers will have no trouble coping with the fact that you are pregnant; others may feel deep embarrassment at seeing the proof that their mother or parents still have an intimate sexual relationship. There may be some resentment towards the baby because they see the newcomer as a definite rival for your time and attention. These reactions are very common and you could try to discuss the situation with them as adults; perhaps by reassuring him or her that you have no intention of remaining heavily pregnant for longer than is necessary and by reminding them of the special place they occupy in the family.

Q CAN MY OTHER CHILD/CHILDREN BE PRESENT AT THE BIRTH?

A This depends on many factors. The first and most important consideration is whether you feel confident that your child could cope with seeing you in pain. Many children find this very upsetting and it may therefore be better not to put them through the experience. If you are having a hospital birth, it would also be difficult to have your child waiting around for many hours. Furthermore, should any complications develop, your partner would have to take the child outside when you may prefer that your partner stay with you. With a home birth, things are easier because you can call the child in at the appropriate moment to witness the actual birth (see p. 144).

Q HOW CAN I GET TIME ALONE WITH MY BABY WITHOUT UPSETTING MY CHILD?

A You could try to encourage a strong, loving attachment between your child and another adult who can occasionally stand in for you. This will not only give you more time for the baby but also enrich the emotional life of your child. You can do this by making sure your partner, a grandparent or a friend is part of your everyday routine. However, you must also make time to give your older child some special attention without a demanding baby around. For instance, you could try asking your partner or another adult to take the baby out for walks so that you can establish a regular time alone with your child.

PREPARING YOUR CHILD

The arrival of a new baby can be a difficult time for your existing child, who may feel left out and so demand more attention. Making plans and preparing your child for the new arrival could spare you the trauma of an unhappy older child. How you tell your child about the new baby can make a difference to how they view the event.

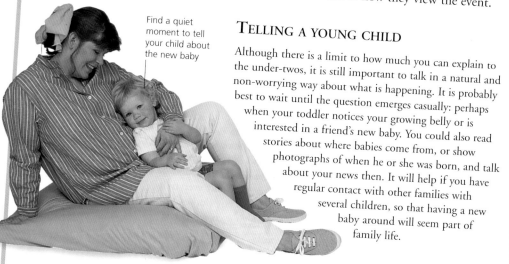

Find a quiet moment to tell your child about the new baby

TELLING A YOUNG CHILD

Although there is a limit to how much you can explain to the under-twos, it is still important to talk in a natural and non-worrying way about what is happening. It is probably best to wait until the question emerges casually: perhaps when your toddler notices your growing belly or is interested in a friend's new baby. You could also read stories about where babies come from, or show photographs of when he or she was born, and talk about your news then. It will help if you have regular contact with other families with several children, so that having a new baby around will seem part of family life.

TELLING AN OLDER CHILD

The older the child, the more you can explain and the earlier you can break the news. An older child may be interested in what is happening to you and how the baby grows; encourage him or her to feel the baby move inside you. You could involve your child in choosing a name for the new baby. All this will help to make the coming birth a family event.

Family and friends can help

Encourage family and friends to make a fuss of the older child. Discuss your concern that your child should not feel that all the attention is focused on the new baby.

Presents

Your new baby will receive plenty of presents, which may make your other child feel left out. When you pack for the hospital, wrap up a gift for your child from the new baby. Ask grandparents and close family to bring something for the older child when they come to see the new baby.

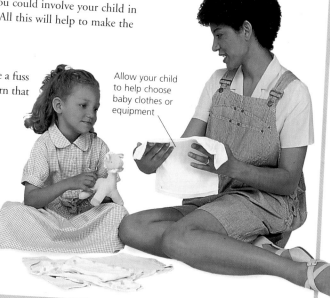

Allow your child to help choose baby clothes or equipment

YOUR CHANGING BODY

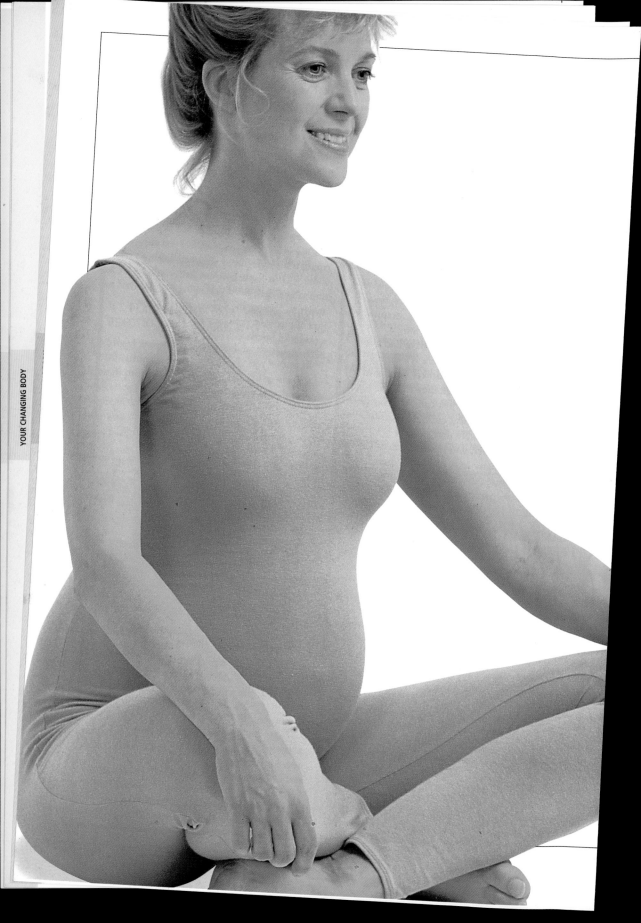

KEEPING FIT
AND
HEALTHY

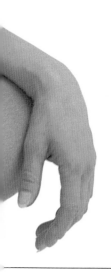

Pregnancy and childbirth place great demands on your stamina and health, so it is important to keep yourself fit and healthy right up to and after the birth of your baby. The focus here is on giving you the knowledge, motivation, and confidence to maintain a healthy pregnancy. To prepare yourself fully for the delivery you need to eat wisely and well, keep supple, and learn how to relax to reduce tension and stress. This chapter discusses ideal pregnancy diets, exercise routines, and healthy lifestyles, which foodstuffs and drugs to avoid, and those complementary medicines and techniques that can benefit you and your baby.

LOOKING AFTER YOURSELF

Q SHOULD I TAKE EXTRA CARE OF MYSELF NOW THAT I'M PREGNANT?

A The more healthy and relaxed you are, the more easily you will be able to cope with the demands of pregnancy. A healthy lifestyle combines many factors: a balanced diet, regular exercise, and plenty of rest. All of these will give you more energy and could mean that you will avoid some of the discomforts associated with pregnancy. For instance, if you eat a balanced diet with plenty of fibre, you will be less likely to suffer from constipation, a common complaint during pregnancy.

Q WHAT CAN I DO TO KEEP HEALTHY?

A Being healthy means eating the right foods (see p. 100) and taking regular exercise. This involves not only antenatal exercises (see p. 106), but also aerobic activities, such as swimming, and going for brisk walks. Remember, however, that this is not the time to embark on a strenuous training programme.

Q WILL MY BABY BENEFIT IF I LEAD A HEALTHY LIFESTYLE?

A Yes, in general, the healthier and happier you are, the better it is for your baby's development. Many things that you eat or drink during your pregnancy can affect your baby, so it is sensible to eat healthily and avoid anything that may be harmful to you or your baby (see p. 98). It is therefore true to say that if you make the effort to have a healthier lifestyle, your baby will ultimately benefit.

Q WHERE SHOULD I BEGIN?

A Take a long, hard look at how you treat your body and then think of ways in which you could be kinder to yourself. If you are a smoker or a heavy drinker, you will need to cut these out or at the very least down (see p. 102). You may have to make a few adjustments to your diet (see p. 100) or plan an exercise routine. Be positive about your new lifestyle – you are not only helping yourself and your baby, but you may also find that you actually enjoy being healthier.

Q WILL MY PREGNANCY AND DELIVERY BE EASIER IF I'M FIT?

A The fitter you are now, the more stamina you will have during labour and the more likely you will be to bounce back after the birth. If you have exercised regularly and eaten well, you will feel more energetic and be better able to look after a new baby. You are also more likely to regain your figure faster. Exercise is also a great reliever of stress; if you feel physically fit and well, you will enjoy your pregnancy more and be less prone to feelings of anxiety.

Q I HAVE PROBLEMS RELAXING AND TAKING IT EASY – WHAT CAN I DO?

A Learning relaxation techniques can help you to unwind throughout pregnancy (see p. 112). Looking after yourself also means ensuring that you do not over-exert yourself, which can lead to exhaustion. This is easier to say than do if you have a demanding job and/or other children, but it is important to make time to relax so that stress does not build up. Taking time out for a massage is another great way to relax (see p. 114).

Q HOW CAN I LOOK MY BEST?

A Pregnancy changes your body in ways you may not expect: as well as your growing bump, it also affects your skin, your hair, your teeth, and even your nails. You need, therefore, to take extra care of yourself during pregnancy (see opposite). Pampering yourself can give you a boost if you are feeling huge and ungainly during late pregnancy. Aromatherapy, massage, and other beauty treatments are just some of the beneficial ways in which you can do this.

Q I FEEL SO HOT AND BOTHERED ALL THE TIME – WHY IS THIS?

A As more blood circulates around your body, you may feel warmer and find that you perspire more. This can make you prone to rashes where the skin creases – in the groin and under the breasts – so keep fresh by washing more frequently. Also try not to put on too much weight (see p. 79), because this will increase your discomfort and make you feel even hotter.

LOOKING GOOD, FEELING GREAT

Hormonal changes in pregnancy can make you look healthy and glowing, or they can have quite the opposite effect.

YOUR COMPLEXION

The extra blood circulating in your body can mean that your skin retains more moisture, is more supple, and less spotty. However, pregnancy hormones can cause problems for certain skins; oestrogen slows oil production, dries skin, and can darken freckles. Because skin texture can change, you may need a different moisturizer. Your doctor will tell you to stop taking any anti-acne drugs during pregnancy. This is important, as these can be harmful.

Greasy skin

If your skin is not usually greasy, don't be too concerned, as this will probably be a temporary condition for the duration of your pregnancy. Use an astringent lotion as part of your daily make-up routine and a special moisturizer for oily skin. If you wear a make-up foundation base, make sure that you use one with an oil-free base.

Dry skin

Avoid using soap, which can dry out your skin by removing its natural moisturizing oils; use a baby lotion, or gentle facial or body wash instead. Using bath oil can help to moisturize your skin, but you should not soak for too long in the bath as this can dry your skin even further.

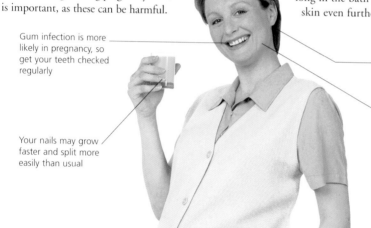

Gum infection is more likely in pregnancy, so get your teeth checked regularly

Your nails may grow faster and split more easily than usual

Your hair may be thicker and healthier during your pregnancy

Your skin will be affected by increased level of hormones and blood supply

YOUR HAIR

Hair grows in a cycle of loss and regrowth. When you are pregnant, your hair remains in the growth phase, which means it may be thicker and possibly shinier. For some women this is good, as their hair looks better than ever. For others, however, it means more unmanageable hair. If you are among the latter, you may find a shorter haircut easier to look after; changing your shampoo to a gentler variety may also help. For several months after the baby's birth, you may shed a dramatic amount of hair as the growth phase of pregnancy comes to an end. Don't worry, you will not go bald; your hair should re-establish its normal growth-and-loss pattern quite soon.

YOUR TEETH AND GUMS

As soon as you are pregnant, make an appointment to see your dentist. Pregnancy affects your gums, making them spongy and prone to infection, so it is important to have your teeth checked and cleaned regularly. You must tell the dentist you are pregnant, because you should avoid X-rays unless necessary.

YOUR NAILS

These may grow faster during pregnancy, or become brittle and split or break more easily than usual. If this is the case, keep them short and wear gloves when gardening or doing the housework.

EATING FOR HEALTH

Q WHAT SHOULD I BE EATING?

A You do not need a special diet just because you are pregnant but you should eat healthily as your body has to work especially hard during pregnancy. It is now known that what you eat can have a far-reaching effect on your baby's health. You should therefore make sure that you have a well-balanced, varied diet and that you eat regularly and often. In the last three months of your pregnancy, aim to increase your daily calorie intake by about 200 calories – the equivalent of a banana and a glass of milk.

Q WHICH FOODS ARE BEST?

A Often you will find that advice on diet includes foods, such as dried fruits, bran, wheatgerm, and avocado, that are high in nutritional content, but are not the foods you would normally eat – or even like particularly. It is far better to be realistic in your dietary aims and eat what you actually enjoy, because it is likely that if you restrict yourself to an artificial (and possibly unappealing) diet, you will be more tempted to go on an eating binge and put on unwanted pounds. Just make sure that you are getting the basic nutrients in your core diet (see opposite and p. 100)

Q WHAT FOODS SHOULD I CUT OUT?

A Try to cut out very fatty foods such as the fat and crackling on pork, fried bacon, and cream sauces. These are likely to make you feel nauseous in the first three months as well as contribute to weight gain. Look out for the fat in convenience foods such as biscuits, pastries, and cakes. Avoid certain foods that carry the risk of infection and damage to your baby (see chart p. 102).

Q DO I NEED TO TAKE EXTRA VITAMINS?

A If your diet is varied and adequate, you should not need to supplement it with vitamins, unless you are a vegetarian (see below). The exception is folic acid, which is necessary before conception and in the first trimester (see p. 12).

Q SHOULD I DRINK MORE FLUIDS?

A As your blood volume increases, you need to increase your fluid intake. Drink water rather than high-calorie fizzy drinks, which are full of sugar and can make nausea and heartburn worse. Even if you have fluid retention, do not cut your fluid intake; try to drink up to six glasses of water each day. Drinking fluid can also prevent constipation, a common problem in pregnancy.

DISCUSSION POINT

HOW HEALTHY IS A VEGETARIAN DIET?

A healthy alternative
Being vegetarian does not necessarily mean that your diet is less healthy. You will, however, need to make up for the lack of meat-derived amino acids by eating a combination of incomplete vegetable proteins that are available in pulses, nuts, tofu, and whole grains such as rice and wholemeal bread. If you do this, your vegetarian diet can be healthy and should not affect your pregnancy. Indeed, you may have lower cholesterol levels than a meat eater and get more fibre from extra vegetables and fruit.

Getting the right nutrients
Your baby takes all the nutrients it needs from you and if you are not getting enough iron, this stresses your body and causes anaemia (see p. 122); therefore, if you do not eat fish, eggs, nuts, and beans, you will almost certainly need iron, and calcium supplements and probably vitamin B12. As well as making you feel very tired, anaemia can affect the baby's growth and your general health. Your body will also be less able to deal with bleeding during the birth.

Q ARE SNACKS AND JUNK FOOD BAD IN PREGNANCY?

A Snacking in itself is not a bad thing (it is much better than feeling faint from going without food for hours) but if you can, you should try to snack on healthy foods. Fresh fruit, nuts, raisins, and raw vegetables are all much better for you than junk foods such as crisps, chocolate, chips, and doughnuts; these are high in calories, fats, sugars, and salt, and although they may produce a fast energy high, they do not contain many nutrients that will help your baby to grow and develop. They may also contain artificial colouring and additives. Of course, the occasional snack now and then will not do you any harm, but snacks shouldn't play a large part in your diet.

Q CAN I STILL EAT FAST FOODS AND GO OUT TO RESTAURANTS?

A Although not as bad for you as junk foods, fast foods can still be high in fat and carbohydrates and, if they are kept heated for long periods of time, many of the vitamins and minerals in the food are destroyed. However, restaurant meals such as freshly made pizza can be nutritious for you, as long as you make sure that you maintain your basic core diet (see p. 100).

Q HOW MUCH WEIGHT SHOULD I GAIN?

A Your weight is not important during pregnancy unless you are very underweight or seriously overweight (see p. 79). What is more important is the growth-rate of the baby; this does not depend on your weight or how much you eat but rather on the efficiency of the placenta and the quality of your food, which supplies the appropriate nutrients. However, you will feel happier if you gain the weight steadily and don't put on large amounts.

Q I HAVE BEEN TRYING TO LOSE WEIGHT – CAN I STAY ON A DIET?

A It is not a good idea to try to slim while you are pregnant, because this is a time when you should be eating a balanced and nutritious diet so that your baby can get all the nutrients he or she needs for healthy development. You will also need plenty of energy to cope with the extra physical demands of pregnancy and labour. Even though you might not want to put on any weight, you will and should if your pregnancy is going well, and this is quite natural and essential.

WHAT BASIC NUTRIENTS DO I NEED?

Protein
This is an essential nutrient which, after being broken down by the liver into amino acids, builds new tissue and is vital for the healthy growth and development of your baby. On top of the normal daily requirement of 45g (1½oz), you need an extra 6g (⅕oz) of protein a day during pregnancy. Protein is found in eggs, fish, meat, cheese, and dairy products.

Carbohydrates
An important food group that gives you most of your fuel or energy, carbohydrates are either sugar or starches. Eat starch-based ones, such as pasta and potatoes, rather than sugar-based ones (see p. 100), because these provide a slower release of energy over a longer period and have fewer calories.

Fats
These build cell walls and are essential for the development of the baby's nervous system, so although you should not eat too much, do not completely cut out fats. The reason why fats are such a dietary taboo is because they contain twice the calories per gram as either proteins or carbohydrates and it is therefore easy to consume large amounts of calories.

Vitamins
Necessary to maintain overall good health, some vitamins such as the B and C vitamins, are not stored by the body, so you need to ensure a daily intake of these. All vitamins are essential, not only for the developing baby but for your immune system, blood production, and nervous system. Folic acid is important in the prevention of spina bifida (see p. 12) in the baby. Avoid eating liver, which is high in vitamin A and can cause problems (see p. 103).

Minerals
Iron is necessary to enable many chemical processes in your body to work and it is essential for the production of haemoglobin in red blood cells. Without iron, your body cannot produce haemoglobin and you will become anaemic (see p. 122). Calcium is needed for healthy bones and teeth and is also important during pregnancy. Zinc is important for healing wounds and for many digestive processes.

KEEPING FIT AND HEALTHY

WHAT IS A BALANCED DIET?

When pregnant, you should eat sufficient protein, vitamins, carbohydrates, fats, and minerals, as well as fibre every day to ensure a balanced diet. The food pyramid (right), shows the food groups and how much of them you should eat. You will be healthier if you limit your intake of saturated fats and sugars (top), and salt (sodium), but eat more protein for growth, and carbohydrates for energy (bottom). The menu (opposite) shows a nutritious daily diet.

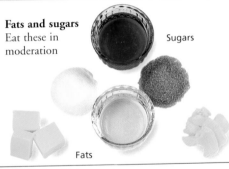

Fats and sugars
Eat these in moderation

Sugars

Fats

Eggs, meat, fish, nuts, pulses/dairy products
2 servings of protein; 2–4 servings of dairy products a day

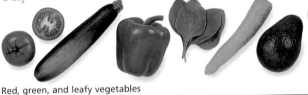

Nuts and pulses

Eggs and dairy products

Fish, meat, and poultry

Fruit and vegetables
4–5 servings a day

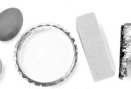

Red, green, and leafy vegetables

Carbohydrates
4–6 servings a day

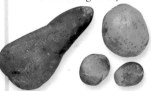
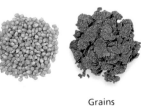
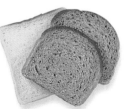

Potatoes

Grains

Rice

YOUR CORE DIET

These are the basic food groups and the quantities that you need for good health during pregnancy. The foods shown above and listed right contain important vitamins and minerals. If you often eat in restaurants or have take-away meals, as long as you make sure that your nutritional needs are met, your diet will be adequate.

Fats and sugars
Eat these in moderation. You must eat fats for your health, but they are high in calories. Of the two types of fat: saturated and unsaturated, eat less saturated fats (animal fat, cheese, cream, and butter) because they are high in cholesterol. Unsaturated fats (poly and mono) such as sunflower, olive, and safflower oils are better for your heart. Avoid sweet snacks: these are high in empty calories.

Eggs, meat, fish, nuts/pulses
2 servings a day of any of the following:
- 85g/3oz red meat or poultry
- 113–170g/4–6oz fish
- 28–57g/1–2oz cheese or 1 egg
- 113g/4oz pulses, grains or cereal

Eggs, meat, fish, and dairy foods are good sources of protein – an essential nutrient when pregnant or breastfeeding. If you are vegetarian, eat tofu, nuts, grains, and pulses.

THE FOOD PYRAMID

Eating sensibly during your pregnancy and afterwards means choosing foods from all the groups shown here. Make sure that you reduce your intake of fats (top) and eat more protein and carbohydrates (bottom).

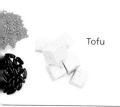
Tofu

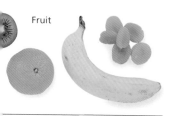
Fruit

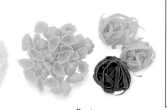
Pasta

A SUGGESTED MENU FOR PREGNANCY

This menu gives you an idea of just how much food your daily diet should contain so that you get enough of the basic nutrients for you and your developing baby.

Breakfast

Cereal with semi-skimmed milk | Poached egg and toast | Fruit juice

Morning snack
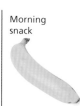
A piece of fruit

Lunch

Pasta with a tomato and tuna sauce | Green salad | Glass of water

Fruit salad and yogurt

Afternoon snack
Milkshake and cookies

Evening meal

Chicken, jacket potato, and fresh vegetables | Roll and butter | Fruit juice

Fruit pie and ice cream

Evening drink

Herbal tea or hot milky drink

Dairy products
2–4 servings a day of any of the following:
- 200ml/⅓pt semi-skimmed milk
- 28–57g/1–2oz cheese
- 1 carton of yogurt

Dairy products provide protein, fat, calcium (for healthy teeth and bones), and vitamins A, B, and D. Semi-skimmed milk contains the same calcium and vitamin content but much less fat than full-fat milk.

Fruit and vegetables
4–5 servings a day of any of the following:
- 85g/3oz vegetables (at least one dark green, leafy vegetable)
- 1 mixed salad
- 1 piece of fruit/dried fruit

These are good sources of fibre and vitamins B, C, and K; some provide potassium and zinc. Dark green vegetables provide iron, magnesium, and folic acid.

Carbohydrates
4–6 servings a day of any of the following:
- 1 slice bread
- 57–113g/2–4oz pasta, rice, or potatoes
- 1 57g/2oz portion of cereal

Starch-based carbohydrates are a source of slow-release energy, fibre, protein, and B vitamins. You need more of these when pregnant or breastfeeding.

HEALTHY YOU, HEALTHY BABY

Q HOW CAN I MAKE SURE I DO NOTHING TO DAMAGE MY BABY'S HEALTH?

A A lot of what you eat, drink, or inhale passes through your body to your baby. It is therefore best to cut out, or down on, things known to be harmful, such as alcohol, smoking, and drugs, and avoid potentially harmful foods (see panel, below).

Q SHOULD I QUIT SMOKING?

A Yes, because smoking and even passive smoking reduces the oxygen and nutrients passing via the placenta to your baby. If you (or your partner) smoke, your baby is more likely to have a low birthweight, and be vulnerable to problems in the first months of life. The risk of bleeding, miscarriage or premature birth also increases.

Q I WANT TO BUT HOW CAN I GIVE UP SMOKING?

A You may find the decision to stop smoking easy if the queasiness of early pregnancy makes the thought of smoking sickening. If not, then giving up or cutting down can be hard. It will help if you have support from your partner or another smoker who also wants to give up, or you could join a "give-up smoking" group, which will offer you support and advice. Start by gradually cutting down; if you find it impossible to stop smoking altogether, then a maximum of five cigarettes a day is less harmful for you and your baby than smoking ten or more. Other techniques to help you stop smoking include aversion therapy, hypnosis, and acupuncture. Do not use nicotine patches during pregnancy to help you stop smoking.

FOODS THAT MAY CAUSE INFECTIONS

Although the chance of contracting one of these rare infections is limited, you will reduce this likelihood even further if you follow the basic guidelines given here.

Listeriosis
Caused by the bacterium *Listeria monocytogenes*, this is a very rare infection. Its symptoms are similar to flu and gastroenteritis (see p. 122) and it can cause miscarriage or stillbirth.

Toxoplasmosis
Usually symptomless (apart from mild flu symptoms), this can cause serious problems for the baby. Caused by direct contact with the organism *Toxoplasma gondii*, it is found in cat faeces, raw meat, and unpasteurized goats' milk. Soil on fruit and vegetables may be contaminated.

Salmonella
Contamination with Salmonella bacterium can cause bacterial food poisoning. This doesn't usually harm the baby directly, but any illness involving a high temperature, vomiting, diarrhoea, and dehydration could cause a miscarriage or preterm labour.

WHICH FOOD	RISK
Liver and liver pâtés	Listeriosis
Unpasteurized dairy produce, especially soft cheeses such as camembert, brie, and blue-veined cheeses	Listeriosis
Cook-chill pre-prepared meals, especially chicken and seafood	Listeriosis
Undercooked meat, especially pork	Toxoplasmosis
Undercooked eggs and poultry	Salmonella
Offal and offal-based products such as haggis and black pudding. Economy beefburgers and sausages made with dairy beef*	*See below

*Although to date there is no clear evidence that there is an association between BSE (bovine spongiform encephalopathy) and human brain diseases such as CJD (Creutzfeld-Jacob disease), it is probably best to avoid these products.

Q SHOULD I DRINK ALCOHOL AT ALL?

A It is impossible to say if there is a safe limit for alcohol, because its effects vary from woman to woman. What is certain, however, is that regular heavy drinking (more than 14 units of alcohol a week) can lead to mental and physical problems in your baby. To be safe, avoid alcohol in the first three months when the baby's major organs are developing. After this, it is quite safe to have an occasional glass of wine or beer with food.

Q IS IT SAFE TO TAKE ANY DRUGS OR MEDICINES?

A The message is simple: avoid all drugs, particularly in early pregnancy, unless your doctor prescribes them (see panel right). If you buy any medicines over the counter, you must tell the pharmacist that you are pregnant. Doctors are cautious about prescribing drugs in pregnancy, particularly in the first trimester. Some drugs must be avoided altogether (see p. 233). Others are considered safe; these include the recommended dosage of paracetamol, and some antibiotics, such as amoxycillin and erythromycin, which may be prescribed for throat and urinary infections.

Q WHAT IF I HAVE TO TAKE DRUGS THAT ARE POSSIBLY HARMFUL?

A In special situations, your doctor may have to prescribe a drug that could be harmful to your baby. This will occur only if the disease for which the drug is given poses a greater risk to you or your baby's health than the drug. For example, quinine, used to treat malaria, can cause miscarriage or premature labour, but the risks from the actual disease are far greater. If you suffer with epilepsy or a thyroid condition, this will also need thorough treatment, or the consequences for you and your baby can be severe (see p. 124).

Q WHY IS EATING LIVER NOT RECOMMENDED IN PREGNANCY?

A Until recently, pregnant women were advised to eat liver as a source of iron. However, we now know that, in addition to iron, liver contains high levels of vitamin A, which in large doses can cause birth defects. The current advice is to avoid all liver and liver products, such as pâté, especially in the first trimester when the baby's major organs are developing. A balanced diet with dairy products, vegetables, especially carrots, and fruit, provides enough vitamin A.

STREET DRUGS AND YOUR BABY

Taking street drugs is inadvisable when pregnant because it exposes you and your baby to a range of hazards. Even the relatively harmless-seeming cannabis can cause problems to your baby. Apart from the direct risks listed below, you also risk contracting the HIV virus if you inject drugs with shared needles.

Ask for advice
Consult your doctor or a help group about the potential problems of using drugs during pregnancy. If you do regularly use street drugs, you must tell your midwife or the obstetrician about this preferably before labour, because your baby may need special care after the birth.

DRUG	EFFECT
Amphetamines	Causes low birth weight
Cannabis	Causes premature labour. Possible risk of chromosomal abnormality
Cocaine	Causes premature labour, serious placental bleeding, and low birth weight
Ecstasy	Apart from the possible effects on you, such as dehydration and personality changes, taking ecstasy may increase the risk of serious bleeding from the placenta
Heroin and methadone	Causes low birth weight, premature labour, higher rate of twins. After delivery: baby suffers withdrawal symptoms, higher risk of fits, increased risk of cot death (sudden infant death syndrome: SIDS)
LSD	Causes birth defects

KEEPING FIT AND HEALTHY

103

EXERCISE IN PREGNANCY

Q HOW ACTIVE SHOULD I BE DURING MY PREGNANCY?

A Unless your lifestyle already keeps you very active with normal occupations such as housework, walking, or gardening, you will probably feel better if you take up some form of regular, gentle exercise during your pregnancy. With a fairly inactive daily routine, exercise such as swimming will help to increase your fitness and stamina and will help you to cope with the workload of pregnancy and the demands of labour. Listen to your body and stop exercising when it tells you to. It will probably not be until the final stages of your pregnancy that you feel too uncomfortable to exercise.

Q ARE THERE ANY SPECIAL EXERCISES FOR PREGNANCY?

A Yes, the pelvic floor exercises (see panel, opposite). The weight of your baby places a great strain on the muscles of your pelvic floor. It is important to strengthen these muscles during your pregnancy to prevent tearing in labour, and also after the birth to aid recovery of the pelvic floor area. Exercising your pelvic floor muscles will help to support the weight of the baby and the womb and help control the need to urinate. There are also specific exercises that help to tone up your muscles and improve the suppleness of your joints, making your pregnancy more comfortable (see p. 108) and relieving problems such as backache (see p. 110).

WHICH KIND OF EXERCISE IS BEST?

Swimming is an excellent exercise because the water supports your bodyweight and allows you to tone your muscles without strain. It can also improve your stamina. Some swimming pools or clubs now offer exercise classes particularly aimed at pregnant women. These are ideal for less confident swimmers because they are done while standing in shallow water. Brisk walking, yoga, and dancing are also good ways to keep fit and supple.

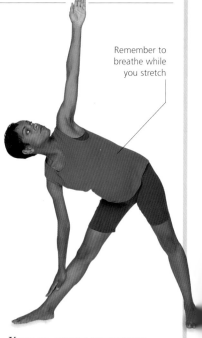

Remember to breathe while you stretch

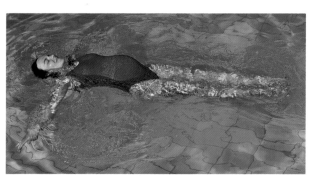

SWIMMING
This can be particularly enjoyable in late pregnancy because you will feel much lighter and the water will keep you cool. Avoid breaststroke if you have pain in the symphysis pubis area or sacroiliac joint problems (see p. 83).

YOGA OR GENTLE STRETCHING
Gentle yoga or stretch exercises are excellent for releasing tension, increasing the mobility of joints, and improving circulation and breathing.

Q HOW OFTEN SHOULD I TAKE EXERCISE?

A Several times a week is ideal but it needn't be the same kind of activity – you could have a varied routine: a swim one day, a walk on another, and perhaps an exercise class or yoga, as you prefer. If you are used to this type of regular exercise, you can continue with it for as long as you feel comfortable, but always listen to your body and slow down if necessary. However, if you are new to exercise, you should start slowly, gradually building up stamina. A little stretching every other day is better than a long hard work-out once a fortnight.

Q ARE THERE SPECIAL EXERCISE CLASSES?

A There are now many classes organized specially for pregnant women. Some offer antenatal exercises, some are for yoga, others are active birth classes. Some pools and clubs also offer exercise classes in water run by qualified professionals.

Q WHAT SHOULD I WEAR?

A Make sure you wear supporting exercise footwear to prevent jarring and damage to the joints. Choose comfortable clothes that won't cause you to overheat. It is a good idea to wear a support bra during any exercise.

Q WHEN SHOULD I AVOID VIGOROUS EXERCISE?

A There are certain times when vigorous exercise is not recommended in pregnancy; these include: if you have previously had problems in pregnancy or your doctor has advised against it; if you have a temperature or feel unwell; in very hot weather. Most importantly, make sure that you do not exhaust or over-exert yourself doing any exercise that you are not used to.

Q ARE THERE ANY PARTICULAR ACTIVITIES THAT I SHOULD AVOID?

A This is not the time to participate in violent or hazardous activities where there is a chance of injury to you or the baby. Activities or sports to avoid include strenuous athletics such as high jumping, or sprinting, and any that require intense training; also, any high-risk activities, such as horse riding and downhill skiing, that could result in physical injury. As always, if you are contemplating doing something you don't normally do, check with a professional first.

THE PELVIC FLOOR

The pelvic floor supports your pelvic organs (the bladder, the womb, and part of the bowels). Pelvic muscles also help to control your bladder and bowels. These muscles can be stretched by the weight of the baby; this causes discomfort and may result in stress incontinence (see p. 120).

PELVIC FLOOR STRUCTURE
Situated at the base of the pelvis, this is a "hammock" of muscles and fibrous tissues suspended between the pelvic bones.

The pelvic floor

PELVIC FLOOR EXERCISES

Strengthen your pelvic floor muscles by pulling and squeezing in the back passage, vagina, and the urethra as if to stop passing urine. Hold.

Slow pull-ups
Pull up and hold the squeeze as hard as you can and count up to ten. Let go and relax for a few seconds before repeating.

Fast pull-ups
Squeeze tight and let go several times.

How often
Practise several times daily, especially near the end of pregnancy, and as soon as possible after birth. As your muscles strengthen, increase the number of squeezes and length of holding time.

Testing yourself
To check that you are doing the exercise properly, try any of the following tests:
- When you are urinating, see if you can stop or slow down in mid-flow.
- Hold a mirror between your legs to see if there is a lift between the vagina and back passage.
- Put a finger into your vagina and feel it tighten when you practise.

KEEPING FIT AND HEALTHY

A BASIC STRETCH ROUTINE

Giving birth tests your physical resources to the limit, and looking after a baby can be hard work, so it makes sense to prepare yourself. These non-strenuous stretching and toning exercises can increase your strength and suppleness; they can also help reduce aches and tiredness.

HINTS ON EXERCISING

- Try to exercise as part of your daily routine.
- Exercise with a friend or partner if possible.
- Warm up and cool down when exercising.
- If you are unused to exercise, start gently to build your strength and stamina gradually.
- If you are a beginner in a class, don't try to keep up with more experienced exercisers.
- Make sure that your exercise class teacher knows you are pregnant.
- Exercise should never be painful or make you feel sick, dizzy, or breathless. If any activity causes pain or discomfort, stop immediately.
- Make sure you do not become overheated with vigorous exercise: overheating may be linked with problems in early pregnancy.
- Drink plenty of fluids (preferably water) to avoid becoming dehydrated.

PELVIC TILT

These pelvic tilt exercises help to strengthen your lower back and abdominal muscles, preventing bad posture.

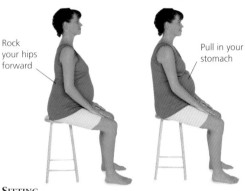

Rock your hips forward

Pull in your stomach

SITTING
Sit on a chair or stool, making sure your feet can rest flat on the floor. Rock your pelvis forward. Then pull in your stomach and rock back on your hips. Repeat.

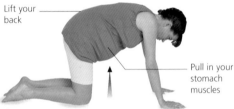

Lift your back

Pull in your stomach muscles

ON HANDS AND KNEES
On all fours, lift your back and pull in your stomach muscles. Imagine your spine is stretching. Return your back to a level position, holding stomach muscles firm.

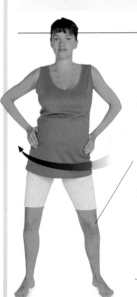

HIPS AND TRUNK

Mobility can be increased by twisting and circling exercises that loosen the trunk area. You may also find these exercises a comforting movement in the first stage of labour.

Bend your knees slightly

HIP CIRCLING
With your feet apart and knees slightly bent, place hands on hips. Slowly circle your hips from the waist in one direction five to ten times; then repeat the other way.

Hold your arms at chest level

TWISTING
Sit on a chair with your feet flat on the floor and your knees apart. Lift your arms to chest level and twist your body to the right as far as you can, then to the left. Repeat several times.

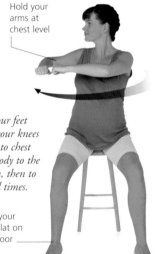

Rest your feet flat on the floor

Leg stretches

The legs carry a lot of extra weight during pregnancy, so stretching and strengthening your leg muscles will be beneficial. The exercises will also improve the circulation in your legs, which could make you more comfortable later in pregnancy.

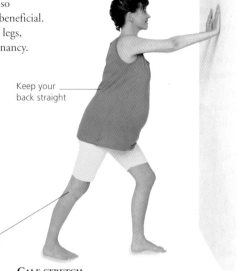

Keep your back straight

Leg strengthening
Stand with your back to a wall with your feet apart. Slowly bend your legs until you feel some pull on your thigh muscles but before you feel uncomfortable. Hold for a count of 20, then return to standing. Repeat this five times.

Keep back leg straight and bend front knee

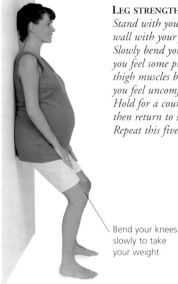

Bend your knees slowly to take your weight

Calf stretch
Stand facing the wall, bend your elbows and lean against the wall, resting your weight on your forearms. Now, with both feet facing the wall, place one foot behind the other. Feel the stretch in the calf muscles. Hold the stretch for a few seconds, then repeat with the other leg. Repeat five times.

Feet and ankles

Pregnancy hormones relax the walls of veins; this slows the blood to the heart and can cause varicose veins and swollen ankles and legs. Do these exercises regularly during the day to stimulate the circulation in the legs and help relieve the discomfort of swollen ankles. This is important for women who have to sit at a desk all day or stand for long periods.

Up and down
Move one foot up and down from the ankle, without pointing the toes. Repeat with the other foot. Perform ten to 20 times per foot twice a day.

Rotations
Make circling movements with each foot ten times one way and again the other way. Keep the toes relaxed.

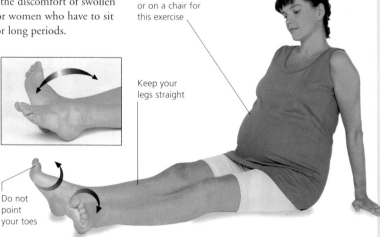

You can either sit on the floor or on a chair for this exercise

Keep your legs straight

Do not point your toes

KEEPING FIT AND HEALTHY

REST AND RELAXATION

Q WHY IS IT IMPORTANT TO LEARN TO RELAX IN PREGNANCY?

A The more relaxed you are, the more comfortable your pregnancy will be and the more you will enjoy it. Your mind and body will work better, you will feel healthier, and your baby will thrive. You will have more energy without tension and stress, because these are physically draining. You will also sleep better.

Q WHAT IS THE DIFFERENCE BETWEEN RESTING AND RELAXATION?

A During the day when you take a rest, or when you are sitting in a chair watching television, for example, you may be physically resting, but not necessarily relaxed: your mind may be active and your body could feel stiff and tense. Reaching a state of complete relaxation enables you to switch off from worries and achieve a calm, positive frame of mind; this will allow your body and muscles to unwind and any tension to ebb away.

Q WHAT IS THE BEST WAY TO RELAX COMPLETELY?

A You don't have to be sitting still or lying down to relax. Taking regular walks or going for a quiet swim can relieve physical tension and clear your mind. Massage and aromatherapy (see p. 114) are luxurious ways to unwind. However, one of the most effective ways to release stress is by learning relaxation techniques (see opposite).

Q HOW WILL LEARNING RELAXATION TECHNIQUES HELP ME?

A If you practise relaxation techniques regularly, you will find that they provide a short break from physical and mental stress and make it easier to deal with day-to-day pressures. You will be more aware of how your body feels when it is tense, and learn how to relieve the tension. This is particularly useful during pregnancy, when sleep may be difficult; relaxation techniques can also help relieve anxiety and therefore help with pain during labour.

WHAT IS THE BEST POSITION FOR SLEEPING?

A good night's rest can seem an impossible quest, especially in late pregnancy when your baby may kick and turn during the night. Sleeping on your front or your back feels uncomfortable and is inadvisable. Sleeping on your side is best; it takes the weight off your back and thus your circulation, which allows an unrestricted flow of blood to the placenta and baby. This position also allows you to try the relaxation technique opposite.

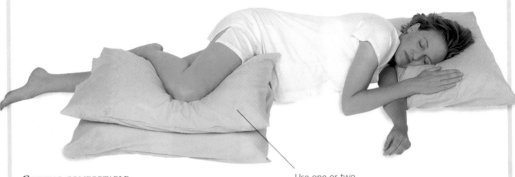

GETTING COMFORTABLE
Lie on your preferred side, put one or two pillows between your legs, and rest your upper leg on the pillows. You may also need a pillow under your bump.

Use one or two pillows to lift your upper leg

Taking time out to relax

The only difference in the busy, active life of a pregnant and a non-pregnant woman is that the pregnant woman has the added physical weight and discomfort of a growing baby. As the pregnancy progresses, you may find it is necessary to take time out to relax mentally and physically. This will help relieve tension and tiredness.

Get comfortable

Make sure you are sitting or lying comfortably. If you prefer to sit in a chair, make sure that your back is supported with a pillow and that your feet are flat on the floor or resting on a cushion or similar support. Alternatively, you could lay your head on your folded arms on top of several pillows placed on a table (see below). You can either close your eyes or leave them open, whichever seems least distracting.

Calm your breathing

Begin by slowly blowing out through your mouth to empty your lungs completely. Then close your mouth, and slowly breathe in through your nose. You will find that this makes you take a deeper breath than you might do normally and you should find that this is calming. Breathing in this way will also help to clear stale air from the bottom of your lungs. Repeat this several times. Your body will begin to relax on the out-breath. Continue in this way until you are breathing in a slow, comfortable rhythm.

Calm your mind

Calming your mind is just as important as relaxing your body, but it does take practice and patience. As far as possible, try to eliminate any distractions from your environment: turn off the TV and any music. Close your eyes and concentrate on steadying your breathing and the way your body feels as you begin to relax. If your mind starts to wander on to familiar nagging worries, gently call it back. Picture a pleasant scene in which you feel happy and relaxed. Explore this scene and conjure up all the details, imagining that you are actually there. Try to do this for at least twenty minutes and then open your eyes and stretch gently to finish the exercise.

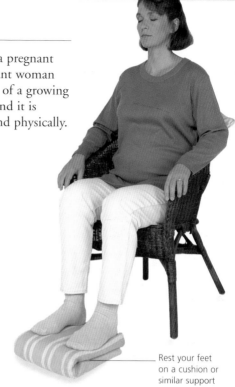

Rest your feet on a cushion or similar support

SITTING IN A CHAIR
If you don't want to lie down, you can practise while sitting in a chair. Support your lower back with a cushion, and rest your feet on a cushion or folded blanket.

KEEPING FIT AND HEALTHY

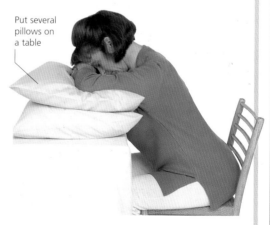

Put several pillows on a table

AT A TABLE
This position, which allows you to stretch out, is particularly comfortable in late pregnancy when your baby is high under your diaphragm and it is difficult to breathe.

MASSAGE IN PREGNANCY

Q WHAT BENEFITS WILL I GAIN FROM MASSAGE IN PREGNANCY?

A Recognized for centuries as a method of healing, massage is an aid to relieving pain and stiffness in muscles. Most importantly, it gives you a great feeling of well-being; it releases tension and restores and boosts vitality; your circulation is stimulated by a massage, which can have either a calming or an invigorating effect. Regular massages during pregnancy will help you to relax and will reduce tiredness as well as relieve any aches and pains, particularly backache.

Q HOW IS IT DONE?

A The muscles and soft tissue are stroked, rubbed, and kneaded gently and rhythmically, usually with the hands, sometimes with specialist tools, which is soothing and restorative.

Q IS MASSAGE IN PREGNANCY SAFE?

A It is safe to stroke most of your body but vigorous rubbing or kneading of the abdomen is not advised. You may find that, except in the first trimester, you are not comfortable lying on your front. Certain essential oils should not be used because they are too astringent (see below).

Q WHAT ABOUT BEAUTY PARLOUR MASSAGES?

A These are fine, but tell the masseur or masseuse that you are pregnant, because some restrictions should be observed. However, a physiotherapist, professional masseur, or qualified aromatherapist will probably give you a better massage.

Q WHAT IS AROMATHERAPY?

A Aromatherapy is the treatment of the whole body with essential oils or essences from plants and flowers to regulate the body and relax the mind and spirit. The oils can be absorbed through the skin either in massage, when they are added to creams or oils, or during bathing; they can also be inhaled from vaporizers. Aromatherapists also value herbs and teas as a means of detoxifying the body.

Q WHAT PROBLEMS CAN AROMATHERAPY HELP ALLEVIATE?

A In pregnancy, aromatherapy can be used to help alleviate nausea, painful Braxton-Hicks' contractions, oedema, and heartburn. It can also be of benefit in cases of tiredness, insomnia, depression, and anxiety. When used in conjunction with massage in the first stage of labour, it can be helpful for its relaxing and calming effects, and for pain relief.

WHICH ESSENTIAL OILS CAN I USE?

Oils used in massage are the "essence" of plants or flowers. Each oil has a different action, fragrance, and sometimes colour. Oils can be antiseptic or antibiotic, astringent and stimulating, or calming and aphrodisiac.

The essential oils recommended in pregnancy
Chamomile, citrus (oils), geranium, lavender, neroli, rose, sandalwood.

The essential oils to be avoided in pregnancy
Basil, clary sage, hyssop, juniper berry, marjoram, myrrh, pine, rosemary, sage, thyme, bay.

Recipes for massage treatments
Mix the following oils in a small jar or bottle and apply with warm hands.

For relaxation 50ml grapeseed oil, 5ml wheatgerm oil, 8 drops neroli, 8 drops sandalwood.

To moisturize the skin 25ml avocado, 25ml almond oil, 5ml wheatgerm oil, 10 drops chamomile, 5 drops sandalwood, 5 drops frankincense.

During pregnancy 50ml almond oil, 5 ml wheatgerm oil, 4 drops lavender, 4 drops sandalwood, 2 drops tangerine, 2 drops geranium.

Relax with a Massage

Massage can release tension and restore the body's natural energy levels. During your pregnancy and labour, a comforting massage can help you relax and sleep better. Lie down or sit comfortably in a warm room. It is best, but not essential, to remove your clothes, keeping the areas not being massaged covered with warm towels.

Where to Start

Your partner should begin the massage with stroking movements, using the balls of the fingers softly but rhythmically, using the hands to work more firmly on tense muscles. The palms can be used to apply pressure, or the knuckles for really tense spots.

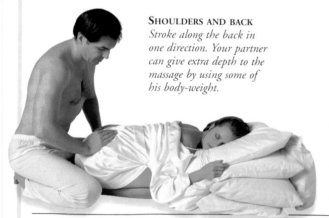

SHOULDERS AND BACK
Stroke along the back in one direction. Your partner can give extra depth to the massage by using some of his body-weight.

EASING TENSION
Rubbing in small, circular movements on the face and around the forehead and temples can relieve tension headaches.

Massage Tips

- Warm the hands; remove jewellery.
- Scented oils, powder, or creams will allow the hands or massage tool to slide easily over the skin.
- Don't knead the belly or breasts.

Massage for Backache

The best position for back massage in early pregnancy, when you can lie on your stomach, is face down on a bed or the floor. Later on, sit on the edge of a sofa or chair and support your arms on the back of a chair, or lie on your side on a firm bed or comfortable floor surface.

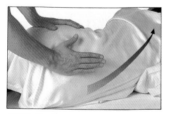

STROKING
Start the back massage with firm, stroking movements from the base of the spine up to the neck, using one or both hands.

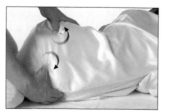

CIRCULAR MOVEMENTS
Gentle pressure applied in circular movements at the base of the spine with the thumbs, relieves muscle tension and relaxes the whole back.

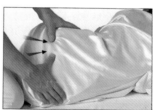

DEEP PRESSURE
Steady, direct pressure applied to either side of the spine is especially good for easing lower back pain in pregnancy and labour.

KEEPING FIT AND HEALTHY

BLEEDING IN PREGNANCY

Q IS VAGINAL BLEEDING A SERIOUS PROBLEM IN PREGNANCY?

A Vaginal bleeding at any stage of pregnancy should be taken seriously. Even if you think the bleeding is harmless, it should be brought to the attention of your doctor so that the cause can be identified and treatment given. Severe bleeding in the early weeks may be a sign of miscarriage or, after 24 weeks, of premature labour and you must seek medical advice at once.

Q WHERE IS THE BLEEDING COMING FROM – ME OR MY BABY?

A Your doctor will ascertain where the bleeding is coming from. Apart from a threatened miscarriage, the most common sources of bleeding are your cervix (the neck of the womb) and the placenta (see below and panel, right). It is very unusual for any blood to come from your baby.

Q SHOULD I BE WORRIED ABOUT BLEEDING FROM MY CERVIX?

A During pregnancy, the rise in oestrogen can cause the cervix to become slightly reddened, causing an "erosion". This is quite common and usually clears up after the birth. Occasionally, there may be light bleeding from your cervix, especially after intercourse. If you have had abnormal smears, bleeding from your cervix may be more important and you should see your doctor.

Q HOW SERIOUS IS BLEEDING FROM THE PLACENTA?

A Bleeding from the placenta may be for two reasons; you may have a low-lying placenta, known as placenta praevia; or the placenta may have come away from the side of the womb, known as placental abruption (see right). With placenta praevia, the placenta is low, covering or partially over the cervix and this may prevent a normal vaginal delivery. Placental abruption is serious and may necessitate an immediate delivery.

Q CAN THRUSH CAUSE BLEEDING?

A Thrush can make your vagina sore and itchy, which may mean that you have a raw area that bleeds, especially after intercourse. It can be treated with vaginal suppositories and cream, although it commonly recurs during pregnancy.

WHAT HAPPENS IF I HAVE BLEEDING FROM THE PLACENTA?

Bleeding in pregnancy is often one of the first signs of placenta praevia. If it is suspected that the placenta is situated low in your womb, you will be given an ultrasound scan to establish exactly where it is located.

What a low placenta means
Early in your pregnancy you will have a scan to check the placenta's position. If the placenta is low, you will have regular scans to see if it has moved upwards away from the cervix as the womb expands. If it does, you will be able to have a normal delivery. Also, if the placenta is very near the cervix, but not actually in the way of the baby's head, a normal delivery may be possible. However, if the placenta completely obstructs the cervix, the baby will have to be delivered by a Caesarean section.

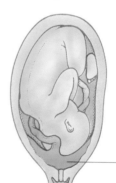

PLACENTA PRAEVIA
When the placenta is positioned directly over the cervix, it is called a major praevia. You will need a Caesarean delivery if the placenta is in this position.

— Placenta

Placental abruption
If the bleeding is fresh (bright red) and you have abdominal pain, the baby is not moving normally, and your womb feels tense and tight, contact your doctor or go to hospital at once. You may have placental abruption – the placenta has partially come away from the womb wall. This is serious because it means that your baby may have to be delivered as soon as possible, even if you are not at term.

BLOOD CONDITIONS

Q AM I LIKELY TO GET A BLOOD CLOT DURING PREGNANCY?

A A blood clot, or thrombosis, is more likely to happen in pregnancy because of the changes in the way your blood clots. When a thrombosis occurs, it is likely to occur in the veins in the calves of your legs. It is not a common condition but there are certain risk factors that increase the likelihood: these include smoking; being overweight or inactive for long periods of time; if you or members of your family have previously had a deep vein thrombosis or pulmonary embolus.

Q HOW DO I KNOW IF I'VE GOT A BLOOD CLOT?

A If you have a pain in your calf or thigh, sometimes with slight swelling and redness, this is a sign of a blood clot. Your leg may also be painful to walk on and the area tender to touch. This can occur at any stage in pregnancy, but more commonly in later months, or just after the birth.

Q IS A BLOOD CLOT A SERIOUS CONDITION?

A A blood clot is painful and may make your leg swell, but its real significance is that part of the clot may break off and pass to your lungs. If this happens it is called a pulmonary embolus; although not common, it is potentially very serious, if not fatal.

Q HOW WOULD I KNOW IF I HAVE A PULMONARY EMBOLUS?

A A pulmonary embolus makes you short of breath and gives you chest pain, especially when breathing in. If you develop either of these symptoms, especially if you know you have any of the risk factors mentioned above, you must inform your doctor as soon as possible. You will need to have a special lung scan and an X-ray test called a venogram, or a Doppler scan (see p. 34), to look at the veins in your legs. Blood-thinning injections of heparin, or warfarin tablets may also be prescribed.

WHAT IS RHESUS DISEASE?

Each person's blood has a Rhesus (Rh) factor, which is positive (85 per cent of the population) or negative (15 per cent). This is a problem only when an Rh negative woman has a partner who is Rh positive – this may result in a Rh positive baby. If the mother's and the baby's blood come into contact during the birth, her body produces antibodies against the baby's blood.

How does this affect my baby?
Your blood is tested every few weeks to check if you are making antibodies. If you do, the present baby won't be affected but a subsequent baby may become severely anaemic because the mother's antibodies will cross the placenta and destroy the baby's red blood cells. This is now rare, however, because women in this situation are given injections of anti-D, which coats the baby's Rh positive blood cells and prevents the manufacture of antibodies.

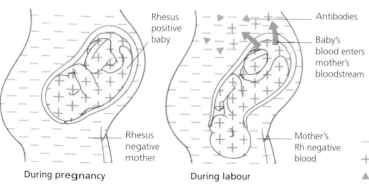

RHESUS DISEASE
Antibodies produced against Rhesus positive blood by the mother during delivery (left), cross the placenta in later pregnancies to cause severe anaemia in the next baby, or even miscarriage.

Rhesus positive baby

Antibodies

Baby's blood enters mother's bloodstream

Rhesus negative mother

Mother's Rh negative blood

During pregnancy

During labour

— Rhesus negative blood
+ Rhesus positive blood
▲ Mother's antibodies

HAVING YOUR BABY IN HOSPITAL

Q WHAT PLANS SHOULD I MAKE BEFORE MY LABOUR IN HOSPITAL?

A There are a number of arrangements that need to be made well in advance of your labour so that everything runs smoothly when you have to go into hospital. Make a list of relevant contact numbers, keep them by the telephone, and tell another person where they are in the event of an emergency. This list should include your midwife's contact number, or the number of the labour ward and your labour partner's daytime telephone number. Keep your hospital notes handy.

Q WHAT OTHER ARRANGEMENTS SHOULD I MAKE?

A Work out your travel arrangements in advance because once your contractions start, you should not attempt to drive yourself to the hospital. If no one else is available to drive you to the hospital, call a taxi or, in an emergency, call an ambulance. If you have children, you should make arrangements for someone to come over at short notice to look after them. They should be prepared to come even if you go into labour in the middle of the night.

GETTING READY FOR YOUR HOSPITAL BIRTH

Plan what you will need to pack in your hospital bag, and make sure that it is ready at least three weeks before your baby is due.

If you leave the packing until you go into labour, you are more than likely to forget something in the excitement.

WHAT YOU NEED

In most hospitals you will need the basic essentials shown here, but you can take other things for relaxation and massage.

Socks

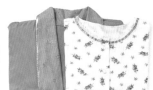

A big T-shirt or nightdress for labour

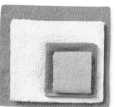
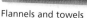

Flannels and towels

Slippers

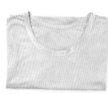

A dressing gown and nightdress for afterwards

Extra items

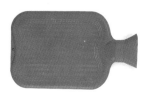

A hot water bottle for backache

A natural sponge, lip salve, water spray, and massage oil and equipment

Essentials for your labour
- A nightdress or big T-shirt
- Socks
- Face flannels and towels
- Slippers
- Dressing gown and fresh nightdress
- Sponge bag with toiletries

Extra items
- Hot water bottle
- Natural sponge to suck on and lip salve
- Water spray bottle
- Massage equipment
- Music for relaxation
- A hand-held mirror

After delivery for you
- Nursing bras and breast pads
- Disposable briefs
- Sanitary pads
- Food and drink to snack on

Q WHAT DO I NEED TO TAKE TO HOSPITAL FOR MY LABOUR?

A You will need to pack a bag of basic essentials (see below). Before you begin to pack, however, ask your midwife for a list of basics the hospital provides in the way of toiletries and bulkier items such as cushions. Assemble the things you'll want for your comfort during the delivery, such as a cooling face spray and a natural sponge to suck on when your mouth feels dry, as well as your usual toiletries for washing and freshening up. You can usually wear your own clothes, such as a large T-shirt or short-sleeved nightdress, during labour. For later in the post-natal ward, you will need a dressing gown as well as fresh nightdresses (front-opening if you intend to breastfeed). Don't forget to pack your sanitary towels, maternity bras, and breast pads.

Q APART FROM ESSENTIALS, SHOULD WE BRING ANYTHING ELSE?

A You may both be glad to have something to distract you during what can be a very prolonged early labour, so your partner could arrange to bring in tapes and a cassette player, games, or playing cards. Remember to bring your favourite massage oils and equipment if you are using them. If you want to record the birth of your baby, pack a camera or video camera. Change or a phone card for the hospital telephone is essential, as mobile phones – which can interfere with equipment – are not allowed. You might consider refreshments for your partner during a long labour, because few hospitals provide food during the night. A change of clothes for your partner is also useful.

WHAT YOUR BABY NEEDS

You need to provide a set of clothing for when your baby is born. The following list is very basic, but should cover your baby's immediate needs after the birth. You will buy more clothing as your baby grows over the coming months (see p. 196).

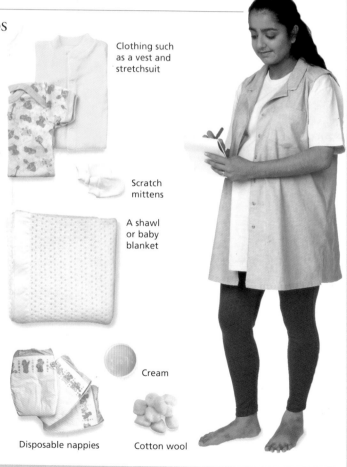

Clothing such as a vest and stretchsuit

Scratch mittens

A shawl or baby blanket

Cream

Disposable nappies

Cotton wool

Essentials
- Two to three stretchsuits or nightdresses, and vests
- Scratch mittens
- A shawl or baby blanket
- Cream, such as zinc and castor oil or petroleum jelly, for baby's bottom
- Disposable nappies
- Cotton wool

Afterwards for taking your baby home
- An extra layer of outdoor clothes or blankets
- A carry cot, pram, or car seat
- A hat

LABOUR AND BIRTH

The delivery room

A hospital environment can seem frightening to an outsider but if you understand exactly what is going on when you have your baby, you can be more relaxed. Your hospital will invite you to tour their Maternity Unit as part of your antenatal preparation. It is a good idea to go along to see the delivery rooms and post-natal wards, and to ask any questions you might have about the hospital's procedures and equipment.

What is the equipment for?

The labour room is full of equipment, some of which can look quite worrying to prospective parents. Below is a guide to the most important items you will see:

■ **Baby's cot** This is where your baby is laid when being checked over by the midwife or doctor.

■ **Delivery bed** Although high, the delivery bed is practical: for delivery it can be raised and lowered, and the end can be removed to facilitate the delivery and stitching.

■ **The resuscitation trolley** This trolley is equipped with oxygen for your baby, and suction apparatus to extract any mucus from your baby's lungs. There is also a heater for the newborn. This equipment is always prepared and available in the event of a problem.

■ **Sphygmomanometer** This instrument measures your blood pressure.

■ **Oxygen** Piped oxygen, if you need it for pain relief, reaches you through a mask.

■ **Gas and air** This is a mixture of oxygen and nitrous oxide that you can inhale to help take the edge off your pain.

■ **CTG (cardiotocograph)** This records your contractions and your baby's heartbeat, and shows them on a continuous print-out.

■ **Extra comforts** Some hospitals supply aids, such as a bean bag, birthing chair or stool, or a rocking chair, for a more active birth.

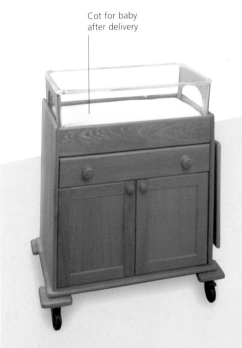

Cot for baby after delivery

Adjustable delivery bed

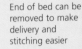

End of bed can be removed to make delivery and stitching easier

A TYPICAL DELIVERY ROOM
This picture shows how most delivery rooms are organized. Your hospital's delivery room may not look exactly like this one but most modern hospitals provide the equipment shown here. Some also offer private bathroom facilities, and there may be a birthing pool.

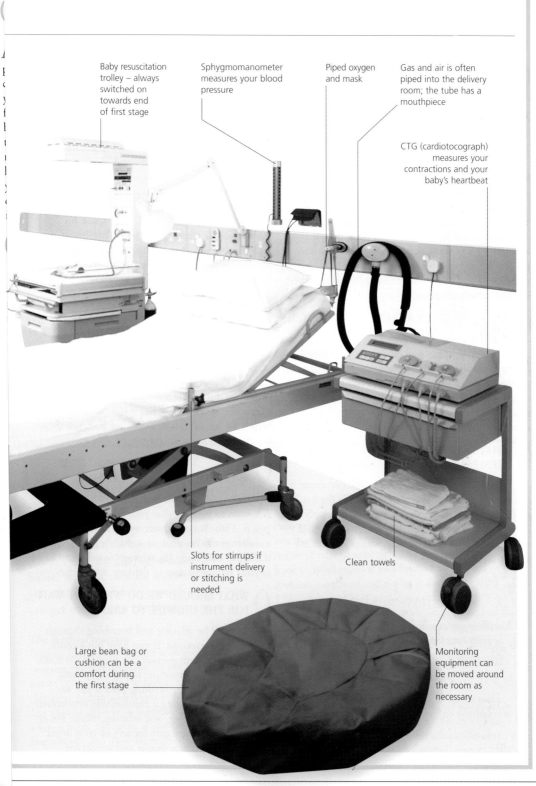

Baby resuscitation trolley – always switched on towards end of first stage

Sphygmomanometer measures your blood pressure

Piped oxygen and mask

Gas and air is often piped into the delivery room; the tube has a mouthpiece

CTG (cardiotocograph) measures your contractions and your baby's heartbeat

Slots for stirrups if instrument delivery or stitching is needed

Clean towels

Large bean bag or cushion can be a comfort during the first stage

Monitoring equipment can be moved around the room as necessary

LABOUR AND BIRTH

WHAT DO I NEED FOR A HOME BIRTH?

Because you have chosen to give birth in your own home, you and your partner are in control of your birth environment and can provide the atmosphere you prefer. There are, however, certain essentials you should provide; ask your midwife for a list.

WHAT YOU WILL NEED

The midwife attending your delivery will bring with her all the necessary medical equipment (see panel, right). Decide where you would like to have your baby; the only requirements are warmth and cleanliness. In addition to some items of equipment you will be required to provide, consider the optional items shown below.

Socks

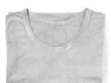

A T-shirt or short nightdress for labour

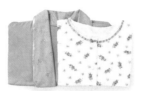

A front-opening nightdress and dressing gown for afterwards

Slippers

Extra items for your comfort

Flannels

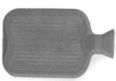

Hot water bottle

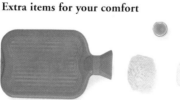

A sponge, lip balm, water spray, massage oil and equipment

Essentials for you
- Something comfortable to wear (a large T-shirt or short nightdress)
- Socks, flannels

Extra items for your comfort
- Small natural sponge to suck on
- Ice chips or cubes
- Hot water bottle
- Water spray bottle
- Lip balm; massager, oil

Items you will need afterwards
- A fresh nightdress
- Slippers and dressing gown
- Nursing bra and breast pads
- Disposable knickers
- Sanitary pads
- Towels

EQUIPMENT YOU WILL NEED TO PROVIDE

Your house probably already contains most of the things you need, but you may want to provide extra cushions so that you have several alternatives for changing positions when coping with contractions. Dim lights may help you to relax during labour, but your midwife will need a bright light for stitching.

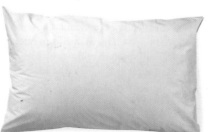

Extra pillows or large cushions

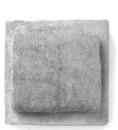

Clean towels

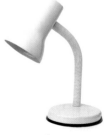

Lamp

FOR YOUR BABY

About three weeks before your baby is due, start assembling all the basic items that will be necessary for your new baby. The main requirements are nappies, warm clothing, and somewhere to sleep.

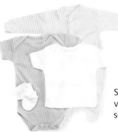

Stretchsuits, vests, and scratch mittens

Plenty of nappies, baby cream, and cotton wool

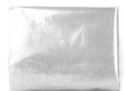

Shawl or baby blanket

Essentials

- Soft, clean towels and sheets
- Nappies (disposable or towelling as preferred)
- Clothing such as two to three stretchsuits, vests, or nightdresses
- Scratch mittens
- Shawl or baby blanket
- Cotton wool
- Zinc and castor oil cream or petroleum jelly
- Moses basket or carrycot
- Changing mat (optional)

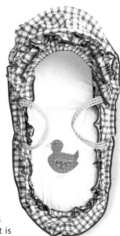

A portable Moses basket or carrycot is best for a newborn baby

THE MIDWIFE'S PACK

Your midwife arrives with a delivery pack containing essential medicines and sterile instruments for the safe delivery of your baby.

Basic labour kit

- Antiseptic solutions
- Blood pressure monitor
- Thermometer; stethoscope
- Doppler sonicaid
- Syringes
- Urine testing sticks
- Oxygen
- Equipment for stitching
- Gloves, scissors

For pain relief

- Gas and air
- Opiate-type drugs such as pethidine (your midwife may ask you to get this on prescription from your doctor beforehand)
- Local anaesthetic

In case of emergency

- Resuscitation equipment for your baby
- A drip in case of haemorrhage

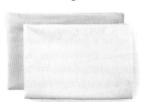

Plastic sheeting

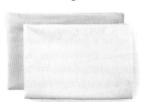

Clean sheets

Checklist for the labour

- Clean sheets for your bed in case you use it, and/or waterproof cover for the mattress
- Plastic sheeting for the floor
- Lamp or bright torch for stitching, if necessary
- Pillows or cushions
- Hot water, soap, and clean towels
- Energy snacks and drinks for you, your partner, and the midwife

For afterwards

- Bags for rubbish disposal
- Clean sheets for your bed

Optional extras

- Bean bag(s) or large floor cushions
- Hand-held or portable fan
- Portable electric heater if the room needs extra warmth
- Music, candles, and/or scented oils to create a relaxed atmosphere
- Camera or video camera loaded with film
- A low stool
- Hand-held mirror
- Birthing pool – you must order this in advance, if wanted

LABOUR AND BIRTH

GOING INTO HOSPITAL

Q WILL I NEED TO INFORM THE HOSPITAL THAT I'M ON MY WAY?

A If you are part of the Domino scheme or have booked a private midwife, she will probably come to your home when your contractions have started, decide when you should go into hospital, and inform the hospital that you are on your way. If you are booked into the hospital or are a part of a Team midwife scheme, try to ring the hospital before you set off so that they can allocate a room for you and organize a midwife to care for you.

Q WHAT HAPPENS WHEN I ARRIVE AT THE HOSPITAL?

A You will be welcomed to the ward, and meet your midwife – unless, of course, she came with you. You can then change into a nightdress or a T-shirt and familiarize yourself with the ward. Your midwife will discuss your symptoms and check the notes and any birthplan you have brought with you.

Q WILL I BE GIVEN MEDICAL CHECKS AT THE HOSPITAL?

A Your temperature, blood pressure, and pulse will be checked, and your urine tested for protein, sugar, and blood. Your midwife will examine your abdomen to check your baby's position, and the strength and frequency of your contractions. Your baby's heartbeat will be checked by a cardiotocograph (CTG) to ensure that he or she is not in distress and that all is well (see below). Continuous monitoring may be needed if there are complications such as a breech baby, twins, a very small or a very large baby, or the presence of meconium.

Q HOW WILL MY MIDWIFE CONFIRM THAT I AM IN LABOUR?

A Your midwife will confirm that you are in labour by giving you an internal examination to see if your cervix has softened sufficiently and is beginning to dilate (see p. 161).

HOW IS MY BABY'S HEARTBEAT MONITORED?

A CTG (cardiotocograph) electronic monitor records your baby's heart rate and your contractions. If your baby's heartbeat is normal and there is nothing else of concern in your labour, you can be disconnected from the CTG so that you can move around. Your midwife will listen to your baby's heartbeat intermittently during the labour.

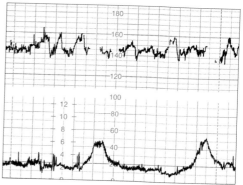

HOW THE CTG WORKS
The CTG monitor is securely attached to your abdomen by two belts. Your baby's heartbeat is detected by ultrasound.

WHAT THE CTG PRINT-OUT SHOWS
The top line of the print-out (above) shows your baby's heartbeat, the lower shows your contractions. These can be interpreted to discover if your baby is distressed.

What is an Induced Labour?

It is sometimes necessary to start labour off artificially. This is known as induction of labour or, if your waters have already broken, stimulation of labour. Induction of labour is usually easier if you have had one or more babies before by normal delivery, and if your cervix (neck of your womb) is already ripe.

Why your labour might be induced

■ When you are beyond 41, or in some cases, 42 weeks pregnant (known as "post dates" pregnancy).

■ If your doctors are concerned that your baby's growth has slowed down or stopped; your baby is not moving well; there is a reduced amount of amniotic fluid; or the placenta is no longer nourishing your baby (placental insufficiency).

■ If you have reached 40 weeks and you have a medical condition that means that an early delivery would be in your interest.

■ If you are at 40 weeks, and you have a vital personal reason to have your baby delivered.

■ If your baby has a condition, such as "hole in the heart", that needs surgery, it is in your baby's interests to be delivered during working hours when the necessary expertise is readily available.

■ If you develop pre-eclampsia, your doctors may decide, for your and for your baby's safety, that your labour should be induced; this may be as much as a few weeks before your baby is due. Your blood pressure will be controlled during the labour.

The procedure for inducing labour

First, your obstetrician will check that your baby is "head down" in your womb, and has engaged low in your pelvis, then will ascertain if your cervix is ripe. You will be asked to return to the hospital at a certain time on a certain day to have your labour induced. When you come in, your baby's heartbeat will be monitored for about half an hour on a CTG machine (see left) to check that he or she is not in distress. You will then be induced by one of the following methods:

■ **Prostaglandin** (vaginal gel or tablets) This substance is found naturally in your womb lining and one of its functions is to stimulate uterine contractions so that labour can begin. If your cervix is firmly closed, your midwife or doctor may put a gel or a tablet containing synthetic prostaglandin into your vagina, which helps to ripen your cervix. This procedure may be repeated several times in one day, or even continued the next day, until you go into labour or your cervix has opened enough for your waters to be broken. The advantage of this method is that it allows you to remain mobile and to eat.

■ **Artificial rupture of the membranes (ARM)** If your cervix is sufficiently ripe, this can be an effective way of inducing labour. Your doctor or midwife will give you an internal examination, then use a long, thin plastic hook to brush against the delicate membranes, which is usually enough to break them (see p. 164).

■ **Syntocinon** This is a synthetic substance fed into your arm via a drip to increase the strength and regularity of your contractions; it is similar to oxytocin, the hormone produced by the pituitary gland, which causes the womb to contract, stimulating labour. This method is often combined with the artificial rupture of your membranes (see above). It is very safe, but if too much syntocinon is given it can cause your womb to contract too much; it can also make your contractions very painful (and sometimes causes double contractions).

Why inductions are not more common

Although inductions are usually successful, labour is not induced more frequently or on demand because there is a risk that you will not go into labour; if the induction fails, then you will need to have a Caesarean. If your labour is induced you are also more likely to need an assisted delivery with forceps or ventouse (see p. 180). An induced labour is less likely to be successful if your cervix is completely closed and your baby's head has not properly engaged in your pelvis.

What to consider

An induced labour may be more painful and take longer than one that starts naturally. You may need to have an epidural; this means that you will be prepared if you later have to have a Caesarean, or even an assisted delivery with forceps or with a ventouse cup.

LABOUR AND BIRTH

THE FIRST STAGE OF LABOUR

Q WHAT ARE THE MAIN STAGES OF LABOUR?

A Labour has three distinct stages: the first starts with regular contractions that open up your cervix, and lasts until the cervix is fully open (about 10cm/4in); the second stage of labour begins when your cervix is fully open, and concludes with the birth of your baby; the third stage is from the birth of your baby until after the delivery of the placenta.

Q HOW LONG DOES EACH STAGE OF LABOUR LAST?

A Every birth is different and the timescale varies, but as a rough guide, doctors expect the first stage of labour to last eight to 14 hours, the second stage one to two hours, and the third stage ten to 60 minutes. If this is your first baby or your labour needs inducing, it can take longer; if this is not your first baby, labour may be quicker.

Q WHEN SHOULD I DISCUSS MY BIRTH PLAN OR PREFERENCES FOR THE BIRTH?

A Once your midwife confirms that you are in labour, you should discuss your birth plan if you haven't done so (see p. 138). Remember, this is to make your feelings clear. If you feel unable to converse because of the contractions, ask your partner to discuss your birth plan with the midwife.

Q WHAT WILL HAPPEN ONCE IT IS ESTABLISHED THAT I AM IN LABOUR?

A Once you are having between two and four contractions every ten minutes, you, your baby, and the progress of your labour will be regularly monitored. Many hospitals use a system whereby the progress of labour is recorded on a graph called a partogram that shows the rate at which your cervix is dilating and acts as a visual guide so that problems can be spotted immediately.

THE POSITION OF YOUR BABY

Your baby's position in the womb will affect your labour. For an easy passage through the birth canal, the best position for your baby is head-down (cephalic) with the back facing your abdomen (anterior position). If your baby's back has turned towards your back (posterior position), your baby presents the widest part of the head (occiput) into the birth canal; this can give you back pain, and also a prolonged labour that may have to be assisted (see p. 180). A breech presentation means that the feet or buttocks are delivered first, and this will also require the assistance of an experienced doctor or midwife.

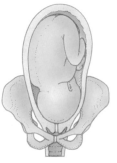

OCCIPUT ANTERIOR
Your baby's head is downwards with his or her back facing your abdomen.

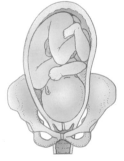

OCCIPUT POSTERIOR
Your baby's head is downwards with his or her back turned towards your spine.

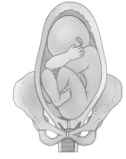

BREECH PRESENTATION
Your baby is presented bottom first, with his or her legs flexed at the knees and hips.

Q HOW WILL I FEEL DURING THE FIRST STAGE OF LABOUR?

A You may feel a range of intense emotions. At one moment you may feel excited and joyful and the next you may feel despondent, afraid, and tired; or you may feel exhilarated throughout. You will probably be stretched to your physical limits, and at times feel that you cannot carry on. Express your emotions and laugh or cry depending on how you feel; this can help you to relax, which can help the labour to progress. You may also be oblivious to your surroundings because your entire being is centred on pushing out and delivering your baby.

Q WILL I FEEL MUCH PAIN DURING THE FIRST STAGE?

A The degree of pain felt varies from woman to woman. The pain usually intensifies towards the end of the first stage of labour when your contractions are becoming stronger and your cervix is almost fully dilated.

Q WILL I NEED PAIN RELIEF IN THE FIRST STAGE?

A This will depend on the intensity of your contractions, also on how your midwife and doctors feel you are coping with the pain; if they become concerned about your progress, they may ask if you want, or suggest that you try, some form of pain relief (see p. 154). If you do need relief, the first stage is usually the best time for this.

Q DOES THE CERVIX START OPENING ONCE CONTRACTIONS BEGIN?

A No, the cervix needs to soften before it can dilate. Labour doesn't always begin when your contractions start. You may have irregular, painful contractions for hours or even a day or two before your cervix dilates, especially if this is your first baby. So you may feel tired, nauseous, and be unable to eat properly while waiting for your cervix to dilate. This is called the "prolonged latent phase".

Q WHAT WILL HAPPEN IF MY CONTRACTIONS STOP DURING THE FIRST STAGE?

A Contractions can sometimes start regularly, but then die away halfway through your labour. If this happens and the progress of your labour comes to a halt for a few hours, your midwife may suggest breaking your waters (if they have not already broken) or artificially stimulating your labour with syntocinon (see pp. 159 and 164).

HOW YOUR CERVIX OPENS

The first stage of labour begins with the onset of regular contractions. This causes the cervix to thin out, known as "effacement". Once the cervix has softened, the contractions cause the cervix to dilate (widen) progressively, so that your baby's head can pass through. Contractions draw the cervix up over the baby's head like a glove, towards the vaginal walls.

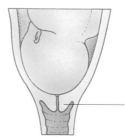

BEFORE LABOUR
The cervix is thick and closed (known as "uneffaced") and your baby's head is engaged.

Cervix is closed

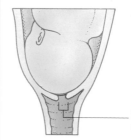

EARLY FIRST STAGE
The cervix thins and softens (effacement) before it can stretch and dilate.

The cervix starts to dilate

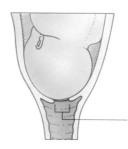

LATE FIRST STAGE
At about 5cm (2in), the cervix is said to be half way towards full dilatation.

Dilatation is proceeding

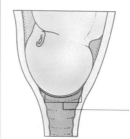

FULLY DILATED
The cervix is fully dilated when its opening measures about 10cm (4in) in diameter.

The cervix is now fully opened

LABOUR AND BIRTH

POSITIONS FOR THE FIRST STAGE

In the first stage of labour, when there is no urge to push yet, you are usually freer to move around and find a comfortable position. Some women instinctively find a position that suits them and stay in this position for the entire first stage. Others prefer to walk around and keep upright as much as possible. Staying upright is beneficial because gravity helps your baby's weight to press down on your cervix which, in turn, helps to open your cervix. If you want to stay mobile, work out a small circuit in the delivery room and place chairs or cushions strategically so that you can stop and concentrate on breathing during a contraction. Try different positions until you find one that you prefer.

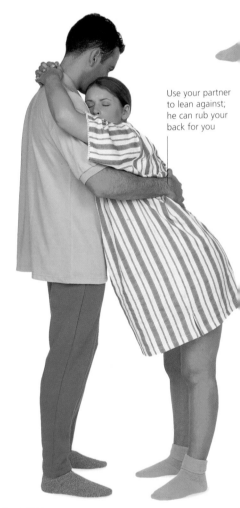

Use your partner to lean against; he can rub your back for you

STANDING
Stand behind a chair, facing the back, and place your arms on the back for support. This can help you to rest during a contraction if you are moving around during the first stage of labour.

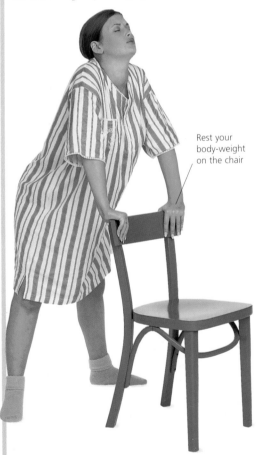

Rest your body-weight on the chair

LEANING
Stand facing your birth partner with your arms around him or her and lean forward so that your body-weight is supported. Ask your birth partner for a low back massage at the same time if this helps.

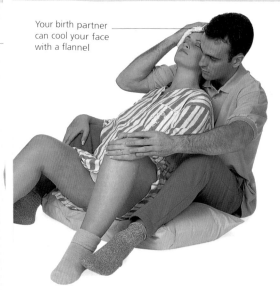

Your birth partner can cool your face with a flannel

SUPPORTED SITTING
Get your partner to sit against a wall or sit on a bean bag or cushion. Sit in front of him or her, allowing your body-weight to be supported. This position can also be used during the second stage.

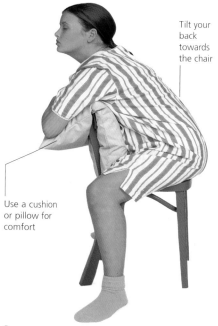

Tilt your back towards the chair

Use a cushion or pillow for comfort

SITTING
Sit on a chair, facing the back, and place your arms over the back for support. Your birth partner can then stand in front of you and sponge your face, or stand behind you and massage your back and shoulders.

THE ROLE OF THE BIRTH PARTNER

Your role as a birth partner is to support your partner both emotionally and physically. Mop her brow or hold her during a contraction; you can also make helpful suggestions, and offer her encouragement and praise. Because she knows you best, the chances are that your partner will take any anxieties or irritations out on you. Be prepared for this to happen, be understanding and try not to take it personally! The following is a list of ideas that you could use to help your partner through her labour:

■ Ask her what you can do to make her more comfortable. She may not know herself, so be ready to make suggestions. Don't get annoyed if she doesn't seem to want to take your advice.
■ Suggest a change of position if you can see that your partner is feeling tired or stressed.
■ Offer to massage her back, feet, or shoulders.
■ Talk her through the contractions and always try to praise her achievement.
■ Remind her how much further on she is than this time yesterday, or a few hours ago.
■ Encourage her to take little drinks every few hours.
■ Remind her to urinate every two hours or so.
■ For distraction, if she is agreeable, read to her, or play a game together.
■ If labour is very long and you are also feeling tired, have some refreshment so that you can recharge your batteries and be of optimum help to your partner.
■ Join your partner in breathing exercises.

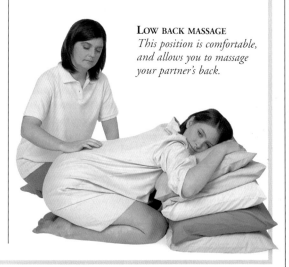

LOW BACK MASSAGE
This position is comfortable, and allows you to massage your partner's back.

LABOUR AND BIRTH

WHAT CAN GO WRONG

Q WHAT PROBLEMS CAN OCCUR IN LABOUR?

A It should be said that most labours are quite straightforward but at any stage there may be complications – minor or major – that mean you or your baby require some form of medical help. Complications include a prolonged labour, unexpected bleeding during labour, premature labour or your baby becoming distressed.

Q CAN LABOUR TAKE TOO LONG?

A There are wide variations in the length of time labour takes; in fact, there is really no such thing as a "normal" length of time for labour. If it's your first labour it can last anything up to 20 hours (although this is unusual). If you are tired, the labour may be speeded up. There are also time limits for each stage to indicate when it seems necessary to lend a helping hand (see p. 160).

Q DOES LABOUR TAKE LONGER IF IT IS MY FIRST BABY?

A Yes, first labours are usually slower than subsequent ones. After you have been through one labour your womb muscles tend to be more co-ordinated, and your cervix dilates more rapidly. There is no known scientific explanation for this.

Q WHY DO SOME LABOURS TAKE LONGER THAN OTHERS?

A Labour can be slow for various reasons. The baby may be quite big, or his or her head may be in the wrong position (its back to your back, "OP" position, or sideways "OT" position, see p. 160). Your contractions may not be strong or co-ordinated enough to make labour progress efficiently, or it may be a combination of all these.

Q CAN ANYTHING BE DONE TO SPEED UP LABOUR IF IT IS GOING TOO SLOWLY?

A If your contractions are not powerful or regular enough, your midwife may rupture the membranes around your baby (see p. 164) to speed up contractions. If this doesn't work, you may be given a drip containing syntocinon (see p. 159). The drip is regulated according to the rate of your contractions.

Q HOW EFFECTIVE IS SYNTOCINON?

A Syntocinon simply performs the task of the hormone oxytocin, which regulates womb contractions, so as long as it is given carefully, it is considered very effective and safe.

Q IS IT USUAL TO BLEED DURING LABOUR?

A It is quite common to have a small amount of bleeding from your vagina during labour. As your cervix opens up (dilates), it bleeds slightly and as the membranes come away from the wall of your womb, this causes a small amount of bleeding. Too much bleeding, however, may suggest that there is a problem and will always be taken seriously by your midwife and obstetrician (see below).

Q CAN BLEEDING IN LABOUR BE SERIOUS?

A If there is severe bleeding in labour, this is called an antepartum haemorrhage and it may be coming from your placenta. If the placenta is "low" (near the cervix, known as placenta praevia, see p. 128) and you go into labour, it can cause heavy bleeding. (If it is so low that your baby can't pass it on the way down the birth canal, you may need a Caesarean delivery. You will have been told that this is a possibility when you had a scan.) Another cause of bleeding is when part of your placenta separates from the wall of your womb, known as placental abruption, which produces pain and bright red bleeding (see p. 128). This is also potentially dangerous and may mean that your baby needs to be delivered imminently, or that you need an emergency Caesarean delivery. Whatever the cause, the bleeding is coming from you, not from your baby.

Q WHAT IS MEANT BY FETAL DISTRESS?

A Fetal distress usually occurs when the blood flow from the placenta to your baby is reduced, so that your baby is not receiving enough oxygen. This may mean your baby will need to be delivered quickly. If it is severe, your obstetrician may decide to deliver your baby by a Caesarean.

Q HOW WILL THE DOCTORS KNOW THAT MY BABY IS IN DISTRESS?

A Your baby's heartbeat is monitored regularly during labour by using a CTG (see p. 158) and any changes in the rhythm will be picked up. If there are irregularities, or your baby's heart beats persistently fast or very slowly, it can mean that your baby is short of oxygen. Another common sign of distress is if your baby passes dark green "meconium"; this drains out of your vagina if your waters have broken (see p. 62). Serious signs of distress indicate that your baby must be delivered quickly and treated if necessary.

Q WILL MY BABY BE AFFECTED IF HE OR SHE BECOMES DISTRESSED?

A Many babies show some signs of distress in labour because the baby's body endures high levels of stress and pressure, but usually the baby's heart rate returns to normal or you give birth to your baby before serious problems develop. Very rarely, a severe lack of oxygen to the baby can result in brain damage; in extreme situations, oxygen deprivation can be fatal. However, your midwife and doctor are trained to identify the signs of fetal distress and to minimize the risk of any complications developing.

WHAT HAPPENS IF I GO INTO PREMATURE LABOUR?

In about five per cent of pregnancies, labour starts before 37 weeks of pregnancy. If your baby is born between 34 and 37 weeks of pregnancy, he or she should be fine and will probably not need special care after the birth. However, if you go into labour before 30 weeks of pregnancy, your baby is likely to be very immature and will need to be cared for in a neonatal intensive care unit or special care baby unit (see p. 214).

Why might labour start early?
Premature labour is more likely to happen if you have had a premature baby before, if you have an infection that is giving you a high temperature, if you are having a multiple birth, or if you are suffering from an infection in your womb.

Is the start of premature labour the same as normal labour?
Yes, often the signs are the same (see p. 156). However, if you are very early (24 to 28 weeks), it is possible that you will only feel low back pain and not experience proper contractions. If you do think your labour is starting early, contact your midwife or doctor immediately.

What can be done to stop premature labour?
Nothing can actually stop your labour once it is underway but your contractions can be temporarily slowed down with drugs called tocolytics. These are not very effective in the long term, and some have unpleasant side-effects, so in general they are not given to you for longer than 48 hours.

What else can the doctors do?
If there is any hint of infection, for example you have a high fever, they can give you antibiotics; if you are feeling very nervous, you may be given a mild dose of a pain reliever such as pethidine. If you become dehydrated, they might also put you on a drip. Often these measures alone can calm your contractions down.

Will the hospital be able to cope if my baby is born prematurely?
If your hospital's special care unit is unable to cope, either because there is no more room or because it does not have the proper facilities to look after premature babies, you and your baby will be transferred to a nearby hospital that has the necessary resources.

Will my premature labour be any different from a normal full-term delivery?
Yes, in general, a premature labour is faster than a full-term labour, because the baby is smaller.

Is there anything that can help to prepare my baby for premature birth?
As immature lungs cause the most problems for premature babies, you will be given a course of steroids 24 to 48 hours before delivery to improve your baby's chances. Steroids can be given to you via an injection or orally; these cross the placenta to your baby and help your baby's lungs to develop more rapidly. If doctors know that you have a high risk of delivering early, you may be given steroids every couple of weeks or so during pregnancy; this is perfectly safe for you and your baby.

LABOUR AND BIRTH

RARE COMPLICATIONS

Q WHAT CAUSES SEVERE BLEEDING AFTER DELIVERY?

A Severe vaginal bleeding after a delivery (called postpartum haemorrhage) occurs when your womb has not emptied completely and so cannot contract down tightly enough to stop the bleeding. Postpartum haemorrhage usually occurs because a small fragment of the placenta has been retained by the womb, or because the womb muscles are too tired to contract.

Q WHY IS POSTPARTUM HAEMORRHAGE RARE?

A Postpartum haemorrhage is rare because your womb has a self-protecting device to stop it from bleeding. Once your baby has been born and the placenta has been expelled, your empty womb contracts down to the size of a grapefruit, quickly closing the uterine arteries so that they cannot bleed excessively.

Q WHAT CAN BE DONE IF I HAVE A HAEMORRHAGE?

A You will be given an injection of a drug called syntometrine, which will help to expel the placenta and make your womb contract down tightly. If even after the injection the bleeding does not stop quickly enough, you may need an operation to clean out your womb under either a general or an epidural anaesthetic; you may also need a blood transfusion.

Q HOW LIKELY IS IT THAT I WILL NEED A BLOOD TRANSFUSION?

A Your chances of needing a blood transfusion are very low indeed, and an obstetrician will only suggest this if it is absolutely necessary, that is, if you lose a lot of blood and your circulation is suffering, your blood pressure is dropping, and your pulse rate is increasing. In certain situations, a transfusion of blood can save your life, so it is unwise to refuse one.

Q HOW CAN I BE SURE THAT I AM NOT RECEIVING CONTAMINATED BLOOD?

A Blood transfusion is a safe practice and carries virtually no risk of transmitting infections such as HIV or hepatitis. In the UK, all donated blood is screened by very accurate (although unfortunately not foolproof) tests. If you are advised to have a transfusion, it is because the doctor considers that the benefits will far outweigh any slight risk of infection.

Q CAN I GIVE MY OWN BLOOD IN ADVANCE IN CASE I NEED SOME?

A This is both impractical and inadvisable. Although you might be able to donate up to one litre (two pints) of blood before you deliver your baby, if you do need a transfusion because of a postpartum haemorrhage (see above), you would need at least two litres (four pints) of blood. It is not possible to give this without compromising your pregnancy and making yourself seriously anaemic.

CAN BEING HIV POSITIVE AFFECT HOW MY BABY IS BORN?

Evidence suggests that your baby has less chance of catching HIV if delivered by a Caesarean rather than vaginally because, as the baby makes its way down the birth canal, there is contact with your blood and fluids that may contain the virus. For this reason, the medical profession also believes that any procedures that can cause contamination, such as fetal blood sampling in labour, are best avoided. If the drug azidothymidine (AZT) is given before and during delivery, it may reduce the chances of passing on HIV.

Physical contact
While you can cuddle and kiss your baby as much as you wish, it is important not to allow any of your blood to come into contact with him or her. Unfortunately, the HIV virus can also be transmitted by other body fluids, including breast milk, so you should not breastfeed.

Confidentiality
If you request it, the fact that you're HIV positive will not be written on your hospital notes and only those midwives and doctors specifically looking after you need to know that you are HIV positive.

WHAT IF MY BABY DIES?

When the baby you have carried for up to nine months and in whom you and your partner have invested all your hopes and dreams dies, the loss is immense and it will be hard to overcome the grief, anger, and depression that it causes. You will probably want to find out why and how this has happened, which is quite normal, yet you must also go on living and planning for the future.

How will I know if my baby has died?

When your baby dies in the womb after the twenty fourth week of pregnancy, this is called a stillbirth, and labour will usually start a few days after your baby has died. You may suspect that this has happened if your baby stops moving, or if you do not feel pregnant any more because any signs and sensations of pregnancy disappear as the pregnancy hormones diminish. You may also experience weight loss because the womb will shrink in size due to the re-absorption of the amniotic fluid.

What causes a stillbirth?

It is not always possible to discover the cause, although a post-mortem may help to answer some questions. Common causes of death include severe fetal defects, or an unhealthy placenta that fails to nourish the baby, either because it hasn't developed properly, or because it has become diseased. Less common causes include Rhesus incompatibility (see p. 129), diabetes, and auto-immune diseases.

How will I feel?

After the birth you will have all the physical effects of childbirth to recover from and, because of the sudden withdrawal of pregnancy hormones, which can cause a flood of emotional feelings, you may feel emotionally raw. While some women find this reassuring because it helps to remind them of their pregnancy, others find that it adds to their distress – be prepared to experience either reaction.

Your recovery

It can take a long time to work through the grief of losing a baby. Life may seem very unreal for a while, and you and your partner will probably find yourselves asking, "Why us?" and "What did we do wrong?" You need to share your thoughts and feelings, but often your friends avoid the subject because they don't know if they will be able to cope with your grief. Perhaps the greatest support can only come from other people who have experienced such a loss. About six weeks after your baby's death, you and your partner should see your consultant to discuss any test results with you and try to answer your questions. Your midwife, doctor or hospital almoner will also be able to put you in touch with a local support group (see p. 232). While you will never completely get over your loss, the intense pain and grief will ease in time.

Your partner's grief

Your partner may have trouble expressing his emotions unless you encourage him. He may even choose to hide his grief by throwing himself into his work or going out more with his friends, which can cause great tension in your relationship. However inappropriate his behaviour may seem, try to recognize what is really going on. Your partner's pain is just as great as yours, and this is his way of trying to deal with it. Try to accept that there are stages to grief that you and your partner may experience in different ways and at different times, and allow yourself and your partner time to work through your grief.

Coming to terms with your loss

Certain rituals and procedures can help you to accept the loss of your baby more quickly and provide you with an occasion or memento by which you can remember your child. For example, you will be given the chance to hold your baby and take photographs, give him or her a name, and think about what kind of funeral you would like. One of the hardest things to come to terms with will be trying not to apportion blame and guilt, because often the reason remains unknown.

The legal position

If a baby is born after 24 weeks of pregnancy, a certificate is given by the hospital so that the baby's birth and death can be registered, and to allow you to make funeral or cremation arrangements. Before 24 weeks, most hospitals will have an almoner or chaplain who can help you to decide on funeral arrangements.

YOUR NEWBORN BABY

The labour is over and you are holding the baby you have dreamed about for so long. But your baby's appearance may be a shock. Instead of the beautiful baby you imagined, your baby emerges with visible signs of the birth, from bloody hair and minor bruising to blotchy, wrinkled skin; it takes a little time for your baby to "smooth out" and become a perfect baby. Your baby will be checked for any problems (see opposite).

WHAT MIGHT MY BABY LOOK LIKE?

As well as being covered with blood and vernix, your baby may be bruised and marked from the birth, especially if a fetal scalp electrode was attached or forceps were used. The skin can be an alarming, dull bluish-grey in the first minutes after the birth, but soon becomes pinker. Add to this a red, wrinkled face, and a strangely shaped head from the pressure of birth, and you have a realistic picture of a newborn. The body's systems are not effective yet, so you will notice blotches, and colour changes that may worry you, but are perfectly normal. Most blemishes will disappear by the time your baby is two weeks old.

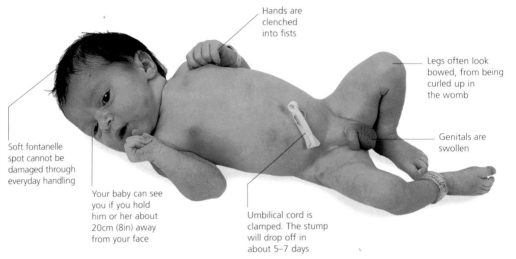

Hands are clenched into fists

Legs often look bowed, from being curled up in the womb

Genitals are swollen

Soft fontanelle spot cannot be damaged through everyday handling

Your baby can see you if you hold him or her about 20cm (8in) away from your face

Umbilical cord is clamped. The stump will drop off in about 5–7 days

The head
Pressure exerted during the birth can distort the shape of the head for the first two weeks. The bones of the soft spot (fontanelle) on the top of the head have not yet knitted together; this will not happen until about 18 months.

The hands and feet
If your baby's circulation is slow to start, the hands and feet may appear bluish, but should turn pink if you move your baby into another position. Fingernails can be long at birth.

The eyes
Blue at birth; true eye colour may not develop until your baby is six months old. Puffy eyelids are caused by the pressure of birth, and squinting is common. Your baby may even look cross-eyed at times in the first months.

The skin
The thick white grease (vernix) that protected the skin in the womb is absorbed or rubbed off. Spots, rashes, and dry skin should clear naturally. Body hair (lanugo) rubs off within two weeks.

The breasts
Your baby's breasts may be swollen and even leak a little milk. This is perfectly normal in both sexes. The swelling should go down within two days. Do not try to squeeze the milk out.

The genitals
Swollen genitals are common in both sexes. A baby girl may have vaginal discharge but this should soon disappear. The testicles of a baby boy are often pulled up into his groin and will descend later.

WHAT IS THE DOCTOR LOOKING FOR?

A doctor will examine your baby from head to toe at least once during the first six days. As well as checking for any physical abnormalities, the doctor looks for signs of infections or other problems.

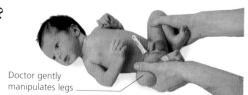

Doctor gently manipulates legs

HIPS
The hips are checked for signs of dislocation by bending the legs up and gently swivelling them.

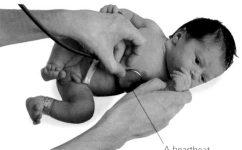

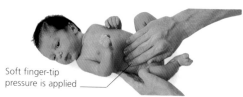

Soft finger-tip pressure is applied

ABDOMINAL ORGANS
The abdomen will be gently palpated so that the size of the abdominal organs can be checked.

A heartbeat of about 120 beats a minute is normal

HEART AND LUNGS
A stethoscope is used to listen to the heart and lungs.

The Guthrie test
Seven to ten days after the birth, a blood sample is taken by pricking your baby's heel. The sample is tested for phenylketonuria (a rare cause of mental handicap) and for thyroid deficiency.

Any spinal problems can be detected at this stage

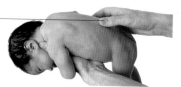

SPINE
The doctor will run his thumb along the length of the back to check that the vertebrae are in the correct place.

WHAT CAN MY BABY DO?

Although newborn babies are entirely dependent on an adult for food and warmth, they are not completely helpless: they can breathe for themselves, cry to get your attention, grasp with their fingers and toes, see your face at close range, and hear and possibly distinguish your and your partner's voice from other voices. Newborn babies are not, however, able to control their bodily functions.

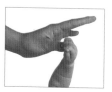

GRASP REFLEX
A newborn's grasp can be tight enough to support his or her whole weight – although you should never try this.

Hands reach out as if to catch hold of something

STEPPING REFLEX
Your baby will perform a walking action when supported under the shoulders in an upright position, feet touching a firm surface.

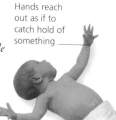

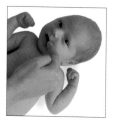

ROOTING REFLEX
Stroke your baby's cheek and he or she will turn towards your finger, mouth open and ready to suck.

STARTLE REFLEX
If you let your baby's head flop back, he or she will think they're falling and stretch out their arms and legs.

Reflex stepping movements

THE FIRST SIX WEEKS

AT HOME WITH YOUR BABY

Q HOW AM I GOING TO COPE WITH MY FIRST FEW DAYS AT HOME?

A It's only natural to feel anxious about your new responsibilities when you arrive home with your new baby. Your midwife will visit you for ten days, to help with any babycare problems. You're obviously not going to be able to run the home in your normal way for a few weeks or months – your main priority is to look after yourself and your baby. Don't struggle on with the day-to-day domestic chores at the expense of your own well-being. Get help. If your partner is entitled to some paternity leave he may be able to help you for a week or two, or perhaps your mother or a friend can stay for a while.

Q MY BABY WAS WEIGHED TODAY AND HAS LOST WEIGHT – IS THIS NORMAL?

A This is entirely normal. If you think of the tiny amounts your baby has eaten, and of the contents of all those nappies, it is not surprising that your baby has lost weight. Newborn babies are expected to lose up to ten per cent of their birth weight in the first few days after delivery. Your baby should regain this lost weight and will probably be back to his or her birth weight by about ten days after the birth.

Q MY BABY VOMITED BITS OF DRIED BLOOD AFTER FEEDING – IS THIS SERIOUS?

A What you are seeing is mucus mixed with blood from the delivery which your baby has swallowed and cannot digest. The best thing for your baby to do is to bring it up. Try to feed your baby again and tell your midwife about the incident. Sometimes the midwife will suggest a "stomach wash-out", which involves her running warmed sterile water through a tube into the baby's stomach to bring out any residue of mucus or blood that may be lying there.

Q WHEN I CHANGED MY BABY'S NAPPY, IT WAS STAINED PINK – IS THIS BLOOD?

A Pink stains are simply the urates (acids in the urine), which a newborn baby passes at first and this is quite normal. However, blood in the urine is very uncommon and should always be reported to your doctor.

POST-NATAL VISITS AND CHECKS

What the midwife does
A community midwife will be given details of your discharge from hospital and she then has a legal obligation (in the UK) to visit you and your baby at home for at least ten days after your delivery. The midwife's role after the birth is to establish that you are recovering from the birth and that your baby is thriving.

Your baby's health checks
The post-natal checks establish that your baby is well or pick up any problems. The midwife asks about your baby's feeding, sleeping, and toilet habits and will weigh your baby at regular intervals (see below); she will also check on the umbilical cord and any delivery marks.

Looking after your baby
Ask the midwife questions about your baby, or about any aspects of babycare, from sterilizing your feeding equipment to what type of nappies to use and how often to feed your baby. Your midwife will also show you how to bath and top and tail your baby if needed.

How often should my baby be weighed?
The usual practice is for your midwife to weigh your baby about three times a week for the first two weeks. Because babies lose and regain ten per cent of their birth weight during the first ten days after the delivery, your midwife may not be concerned with the baby's weight gain as long as he or she is feeding well, until after ten days.

Should my baby be given vitamin K?
Yes, because newborn babies are low in vitamin K and this helps blood clot and protects against haemorrhage (especially into the brain). Vitamin K can be given by mouth or injection but if you had a forceps, ventouse or Caesarean delivery, or gave birth prematurely, your baby should be given the injection. Earlier concerns of a link between the vitamin K injection and childhood cancer are almost certainly unfounded.

Q MY BABY'S BOWEL MOTIONS ARE GREENISH-BLACK – IS ANYTHING WRONG?

A Your baby is completely normal! The first few bowel movements are made up of "meconium", the sticky, dark substance that lined your baby's bowel during the pregnancy and is now being excreted. This may take up to 48 hours to pass through, after which your baby's motions will be more solid, and yellow in colour.

Q HOW OFTEN SHOULD MY BABY PASS URINE AND EMPTY HIS OR HER BOWELS?

A How much a newborn baby urinates can vary considerably but as long as it happens at least once every 24 hours all is well. Usually, however, because their bladders are so tiny, newborns tend to urinate every hour. Bowel movements also vary greatly but again should occur at least once a day. It may be that your baby had a big bowel movement just before, during, or just after birth and so may not need to have another bowel movement for some time. The first bowel movement is significant because it confirms that the anus is open. The same goes for urinating: it shows that the baby's kidneys, bladder, and all the other plumbing are working properly.

Q WHEN WILL MY BABY SETTLE INTO A ROUTINE?

A You will end up feeling very frustrated if you try to make your baby conform to a set pattern at this stage. Just go with the flow in these early days, taking each very different day as it comes. Old-fashioned ideas of imposing discipline and a routine on very young babies serve no real purpose and usually fail. Babies have different sleep patterns (see p. 200); some sleep for long periods of time, others sleep fitfully, but after a few weeks or months a sleeping and waking pattern will gradually emerge.

HANDLING YOUR NEWBORN

You may be afraid to handle your newborn baby at first because he or she seems so small. The important thing is to support the baby's head, because the neck muscles are still quite weak. Because it is reassuring and helps you to develop a relationship with your baby, talk to your baby when changing a nappy or giving a bath. You will soon gain enough confidence to be able to relax when handling your baby.

PICKING UP YOUR BABY

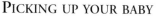

Carefully slide your hands under your baby's head and bottom

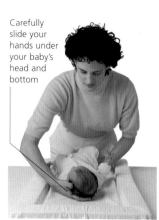

Gently support your baby's head in your hand

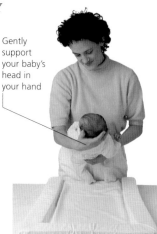

Cuddling your baby will stop him or her crying

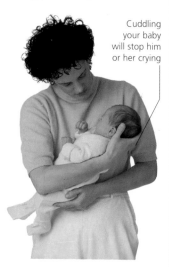

1 Lift your baby by placing one hand under the head and one under the bottom.

2 Lift slowly and gently while supporting your baby's body and head with each hand.

3 Turn your baby so that the head and the back are supported by your arms.

THE FIRST SIX WEEKS

CARING FOR YOUR BABY

Q HOW CAN I MAKE SURE THAT MY BABY IS COMFORTABLE AND CONTENT?

A Your baby has simple, but time-consuming needs during the first few weeks of life. Making sure that your baby is warm, comfortable, and satisfied will keep him or her content. You'll be feeding and holding your baby constantly, and spending a lot of time changing nappies after feeds, when your baby wakes, and before your baby sleeps. These basic tasks can be enjoyable for both of you if you play games, chat to, and cuddle your baby as you do them.

Q I DON'T LIKE TOUCHING MY BABY'S CORD, DO I HAVE TO CLEAN IT?

A Your baby's cord will dry up, wither, and drop off naturally about five to seven days after the birth. However, keep the cord as dry as possible, even if you do not actively clean it: make sure that the nappy isn't covering the cord and dry the cord thoroughly after bathing your baby. Some midwives recommend applying surgical spirit or antiseptic powder, or give you sterile swabs to clean it. If the cord or navel area gets swollen, red, smelly, or weepy, tell your midwife or doctor.

ESSENTIALS FOR YOUR NEWBORN BABY

Preparing for the arrival of your baby can be one of the most enjoyable parts of your pregnancy, as you shop for clothes and equipment. Remember, when buying baby clothes, that your baby will grow quickly, so buy only a few of the smaller sized items to begin with. Below are some suggestions for the basic items you will need.

PRACTICAL ITEMS

- Several packs of disposable nappies (or 2 dozen towelling nappies with plastic pants and liners, 2 nappy buckets and sterilizing powder, and some safety pins)
- Barrier cream (e.g., zinc and castor oil or petroleum jelly)
- Plastic changing mat
- Cotton wool
- Baby soap/shampoo/liquid soap/baby lotion/oil (for dry skin)
- Waterproof apron
- Baby bath
- Sponge/flannel
- Large, soft towel
- Baby brush

Shaped fabric nappy

Cotton wool   Cream   Disposable nappy

SLEEPING

- Cot or Moses basket
- Cot and mattress (when your baby is older)
- 4 cotton sheets for cot/pram
- 2 soft, lightweight blankets
- Baby alarm (optional)

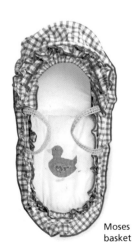

Moses basket

CLOTHES

Choose machine-washable clothes in natural fabrics
- 4 stretchsuits/rompers
- 3 vests/bodysuits
- Light cotton nighties (if too hot to sleep in bodysuit; makes it easier to change nappies)
- 2 pairs of socks and bootees
- Shawl (optional)
- Scratch mittens, bibs
- In winter: cardigan, woolly hat
In summer: light summer hat

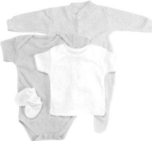

Stretchsuits, vests, and mittens

Q WHAT TYPES OF NAPPIES ARE AVAILABLE AND WHICH SHOULD I CHOOSE?

A There are two types of nappy: fabric, which you can wash and are reusable; or disposable. Disposable nappies are more costly over a period of time, but are convenient to use. There is a wide range available for boys or girls and from newborn to toddler sizes. Occasionally, babies are sensitive to disposables and develop a mild rash, so you may need to change your brand of nappy. Although fabric nappies involve more work, they do work out cheaper in the long run. And you can choose between buying terry towelling squares or shaped fabric nappies. You will need to buy 20 or more and will have to wash and sterilize them after each use, using special nappy-cleaning powder and nappy buckets to soak the fabric nappies in.

Q DO I NEED TO USE BARRIER CREAM EACH TIME I CHANGE A NAPPY?

A After the birth, using a gentle barrier cream, like petroleum jelly, can make it easier to clean off meconium (see p. 62) from your baby's bottom. After a few days, when your baby stops passing meconium, you may need to use a small amount of cream if your baby develops a rash or soreness.

Q HOW DO I KNOW IF MY BABY IS WARM ENOUGH?

A The hands and feet are cooler than the rest of the body so, to find out if your baby is cold, feel the chest, head, or back of neck. If the skin is cool, it is better to put an extra layer of clothes on your baby rather than turn up the heating, because these can be easily removed if your baby overheats.

CHANGING YOUR BABY'S NAPPY

Keeping everything you need in one place will make the task much easier. When putting on a fresh disposable nappy, avoid touching the front of the nappy if you have cream or oil on your fingers as this may stop the tabs from sticking.

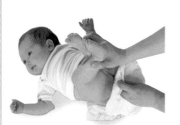

1 Open the soiled nappy and remove any faeces with a clean part of the nappy, then discard.

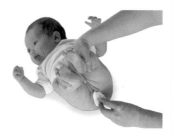

2 Clean the bottom: wipe in the skin creases using several pieces of wet cotton wool. Dry carefully.

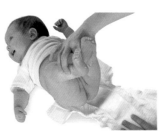

3 Lay the new nappy flat beneath your baby, and line the top up with your baby's waist.

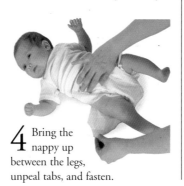

4 Bring the nappy up between the legs, unpeal tabs, and fasten.

Cleaning a boy
Wipe gently, don't drag on the skin of the penis or pull the foreskin back.

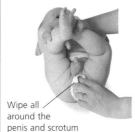

Wipe all around the penis and scrotum

Cleaning a girl
To prevent the spread of bacteria from the anus to the vagina, always wipe from the front to the back.

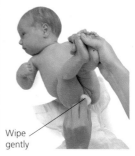

Wipe gently

197

BATHING AND DRESSING YOUR BABY

With a little care and organization, washing your baby can be a playful experience, and dressing your baby in snug-fitting clothes can be a simple procedure. Gather everything you need before you start because you should never leave your baby unattended (see p. 196). If you still have to move away to get something or, for example, to answer the telephone, take your baby with you. As you clean and change your baby, always remember to keep talking to and cuddling him or her.

TOPPING AND TAILING YOUR BABY

Your baby's face, hands, and bottom are prone to irritation from sweat, urine, and soiling, and must be cleaned daily. Topping and tailing enables you to clean these areas without giving your baby a full bath. To reduce the risk of infection, start with the face and finish with the bottom.

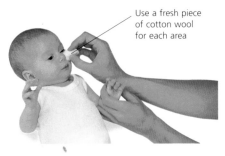

Use a fresh piece of cotton wool for each area

1 Cool some boiled water. Wipe each eye from the corner out, using a new piece of cotton wool for each eye. Wipe over and behind, but not inside, the ears, and then clean the face and around the nose.

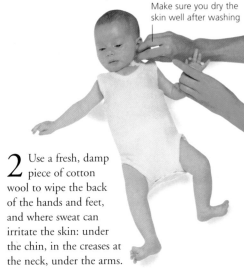

Make sure you dry the skin well after washing

2 Use a fresh, damp piece of cotton wool to wipe the back of the hands and feet, and where sweat can irritate the skin: under the chin, in the creases at the neck, under the arms.

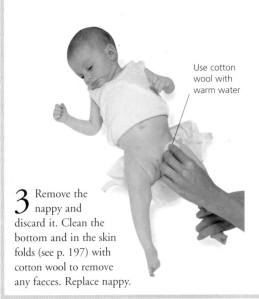

Use cotton wool with warm water

3 Remove the nappy and discard it. Clean the bottom and in the skin folds (see p. 197) with cotton wool to remove any faeces. Replace nappy.

Cleaning the cord

Using cotton wool and surgical spirit, clean in the creases around the stump. Dry with a fresh piece of cotton wool.

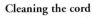

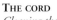

Don't pull on the stump or try to remove it

THE CORD
Cleaning the stump will help to prevent any infection.

BATHING YOUR BABY

Put cold, then hot water in the bath; test the water temperature with your elbow: it should be warm, not hot. With the vest on, clean the face and neck (see opposite). Remove the vest to wash the hair, and remove the nappy to bathe your baby.

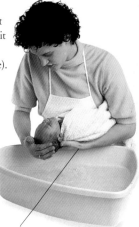

1 With your baby wrapped in a towel, lower the head over the tub and gently pour water over your baby's hair. Gently rub shampoo into the hair and rinse away with water, avoiding the face.

Support your baby's body with your arm, and the head and neck with your hand

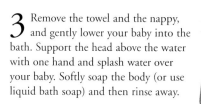

2 A baby can lose a lot of heat through his or her head, so dry your baby's head immediately by gently patting it with a towel.

Comfort your baby by talking constantly to him or her

3 Remove the towel and the nappy, and gently lower your baby into the bath. Support the head above the water with one hand and splash water over your baby. Softly soap the body (or use liquid bath soap) and then rinse away.

Keep the head above the water

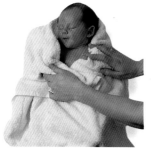

4 Place your baby in a soft, dry towel. Pat your baby dry, making sure there is no dampness between the skin creases. If you wish, apply cream or talcum powder but not both.

DRESSING YOUR BABY

You can ease your baby gently into close-fitting clothes, such as vests or bodysuits, by stretching and rolling the neck and arm openings. Babies often cry while being dressed, but this is usually because they don't like to feel the air on their skin. Never lay your baby near the edge of a surface because he or she could roll off.

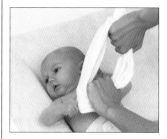

1 Roll the vest up and pull the neck wide so that it is ready to slip over your baby's head.

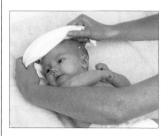

2 Bring the vest over the head, making sure that it doesn't drag over your baby's face.

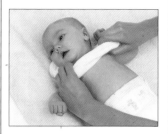

3 Stretch the armholes and guide the arms through; roll the vest down over the body.

THE FIRST SIX WEEKS

BREASTFEEDING AND YOU

Q CAN I MAKE BREASTFEEDING EASIER OR LESS DEMANDING?

A Breastfeeding can present physical and practical problems. Expressing your milk and knowing how to deal with sore breasts can help.

Q WHY MIGHT I WANT TO EXPRESS MY MILK?

A Expressing breast milk into a bottle gives you flexibility, allowing you to store your milk and enabling your partner or other carer to help with feeds. For a baby in special care, expressed milk ensures that the mother's natural immunity is passed on via her breast milk. Expressed milk is useful when you and your baby cannot be together: if you go out for an evening, or later on when you return to work.

Q WHEN IS THE BEST TIME TO EXPRESS – BEFORE OR AFTER FEEDING MY BABY?

A It is best to express milk between feeds. If you express before feeding, there may not be enough to satisfy your baby, and if you express afterwards there may not be much milk left. Or you could feed with one breast entirely and express the milk from the other one.

Q HOW DO I STORE EXPRESSED MILK?

A You can store it the same way as formula: in the fridge or the freezer. The milk keeps for up to 72 hours in the fridge; you should not "top up" an existing supply. It will keep in the freezer for up to six months, stored in ice cube trays or bags.

HOW TO EXPRESS YOUR MILK

There are two ways to express your breast milk: either with your hands or by using a pump (see below). Expressing by hand is fairly easy and painless but very slow, whereas a pump is often quicker and less tiring. Hand expressing may help to relieve sore, engorged breasts, and may be less painful than expressing by pump.

By hand
Wash your hands, have a sterile bowl ready, support your breast in one hand and massage around the entire breast, including the underside, at least ten times. Stroking and gentle pressure towards the areola squeezes the milk out through the nipple.

By pump
Pumps can be manual or battery-operated. All pumps vary slightly but work on the same principle: a funnel forms a seal over your nipple, you then pump the milk out by suction. The milk collects in the bottle attached to the pump.

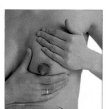

MASSAGE FIRST
In order to encourage the flow of milk though the milk ducts, massage around the entire breast at least ten times.

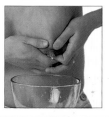

SQUEEZE LAST
Squeeze areola with the thumbs and forefingers together, while pressing backwards; the milk should begin to spurt out. Continue this action for several minutes.

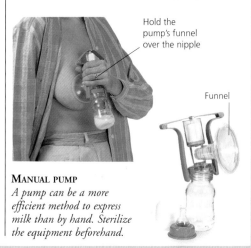

Hold the pump's funnel over the nipple

Funnel

MANUAL PUMP
A pump can be a more efficient method to express milk than by hand. Sterilize the equipment beforehand.

IF YOU HAVE PROBLEMS

If you have any difficulties with your breasts or breastfeeding, you should seek professional help as soon as possible. Never struggle on alone or give up – persevere, because it will be worth it. You could ask your midwife or health visitor for advice or talk to a support group (see p. 232).

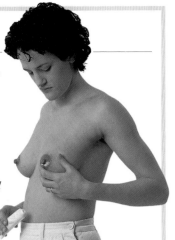

CARING FOR YOUR BREASTS

Let the air get to your nipples often, and wash your breasts every day – but don't use soap, which can be drying. Gently pat yourself dry. Support your breasts with a good maternity bra, and wear it day and night in the early weeks. If milk leaks between feeds (and this is common), buy some breast pads and wear them inside your bra for protection. Change the pads frequently.

LEAKING BREASTS
A disposable breast pad will absorb any drips and small leaks.

Front-opening maternity bra

Engorgement
The production of milk is a finely tuned "supply and demand" process, but when your milk first comes in, it takes a while to achieve a balance. Your breasts may become hard, swollen, and sore (known as engorgement) because they are producing too much milk; this can raise your temperature and make you feel feverish and weepy.

Can expressing milk relieve engorgement?
If your breasts are engorged, nursing is difficult for your baby and painful for you. Expressing large amounts of milk is not the answer because your body will keep producing milk to this capacity. However, expressing a small amount of milk can bring relief. You could also try applying alternate warm and cold cloths, or use the showerhead to spray warm and then cold water on your breasts. A pain reliever such as paracetamol may help.

NIPPLE CREAM
A calendula-based cream may help to relieve the soreness.

Sore and cracked nipples
It is normal to have tender nipples for the first few days, as they take time to toughen up. If your baby isn't latching on properly (see p. 202), he or she may be chewing your nipples and damaging soft tissue, even making them bleed. If you are not in too much pain, it is safe to continue feeding. Your milk contains natural antiseptics, so after every feed, rub some of your milk around the nipple and allow it to dry naturally. You may need to use a special nipple cream, such as a calendula cream; consult your midwife or doctor.

Breast inflammation
If one or both breasts become red, patchy, and very sore, you may have a condition called mastitis, when the flow of milk is blocked, causing stagnation. The milk and surrounding tissue may become infected by bacteria that have entered the milk ducts through your nipple.

Can breast inflammation be relieved?
In its early stages, this condition may respond to antibiotics and pain-relieving drugs. It is important to continue breastfeeding in order to empty the breasts and relieve pressure. If you have a high temperature and feel nauseous and dizzy, and have a hot, firm lump in your breast, this is an abscess; you will need to go to hospital to have the lump drained.

Pain-relieving drugs and breastfeeding
It is safe to take most drugs that are based on paracetamol, because only a very small amount passes across in the milk and reaches the baby. However, aspirin is best avoided because it has been linked to a rare condition (Reye's syndrome) that can affect babies.

BEGINNING BOTTLE-FEEDING

Q I HAVE DECIDED NOT TO BREASTFEED, DO I NEED TO TELL MY MIDWIFE?

A If you are having a hospital birth, tell your midwife who will advise hospital staff. They will provide bottle-feeding equipment and formula and show you how to use it. However, your midwife will not supply bottle-feeding equipment for a home birth; she will discuss this with you before the birth and advise you to buy the equipment and formula.

Q WHICH FORMULA SHOULD I BUY?

A Most of the wide variety of baby formulas now available are based on cows' milk and contain vitamins and minerals. If you don't want your baby to have animal products or your baby develops an allergy to cows' milk, there are soya milk formulas. Dry powder formulas are cheaper, but ready-made formulas are more convenient.

Q WHY IS IT SO IMPORTANT TO CLEAN AND STERILIZE ALL THE EQUIPMENT?

A Clean equipment is crucial because milk is an ideal breeding ground for the bacteria that cause gastroenteritis, a disease that can be life-threatening in a young baby. You must sterilize everything that comes into contact with the feed.

Q HOW DO I MAKE SURE THAT THE EQUIPMENT IS STERILE?

A Wash everything in warm, soapy water. Scrub bottle rims, clean right to the bottom of the bottles, and turn the teats inside out to wash them. If milk builds up inside the teats, use salt to rub it away, and rinse well. Then sterilize the equipment, either by placing the bottles and teats in a steamer, immersing them in sterilizing fluid, or microwaving them. Keep the equipment below water level, and remove any air bubbles. Replace the fluid daily.

WHAT EQUIPMENT DO I NEED?

Essential equipment for bottle-feeding includes four to six bottles and teats. To make a feed you need a measuring jug, a funnel, a plastic spoon, and a plastic knife for levelling off the formula. To sterilize equipment you need a bottle brush, salt, and either sterilizing fluid/tablets, or a steam sterilizer.

Feeding equipment

Cap

Ring and disc

Teat

TYPES OF BOTTLE AND TEATS

Bottles are usually made of plastic. One system consists of disposable bags that fit inside a plastic tube. Teats can be made of latex or silicone and come in several shapes: experiment to find the one that suits your baby best.

Wide-necked bottle with silicone teat

With this system, only the teat needs to be sterilized

250ml (8oz) bottle

125ml (4oz) bottle

Disposable plastic bottle liner

Other equipment

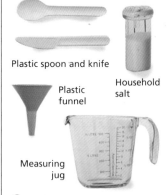

Bottle brush

Plastic spoon and knife

Plastic funnel

Household salt

Measuring jug

CARING FOR THE EQUIPMENT

Remember to keep all equipment scrupulously clean. Rub the inside of teats with salt, clean bottles with a bottle brush. Sterilize all equipment. Plastic or glass is best.

HOW DO I MAKE UP A FEED?

When making up your baby's feed, it is important to follow the directions on the can (or packet) exactly. Do not add extra scoops, or dilute the formula further, or add cereals to your baby's feed. To do so changes the specific concentration and could lead to obesity or even serious illness in your baby. Always use previously boiled tap water.

REMEMBER

- *Read the instructions on the formula can (or packet) carefully and follow them closely.*
- *Wash your hands before beginning.*
- *If you become distracted when measuring the formula, throw the milk away and start again.*
- *Don't keep unfinished feed.*
- *Don't reheat unused milk: this is a dangerous source of bacteria.*
- *Don't warm up milk in a microwave oven.*

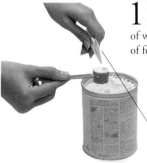

1 Fill the jug with the correct amount of water. Open the can of formula and use the scoop provided to measure out the exact amount.

Level each scoop with the back of the knife

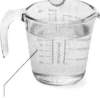

Level scoop

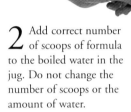

2 Add correct number of scoops of formula to the boiled water in the jug. Do not change the number of scoops or the amount of water.

Boiled tap (not mineral) water

Use a plastic spoon to stir

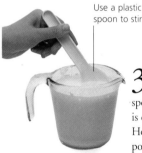

3 Stir the formula well with a plastic spoon until the powder is completely dissolved. Hot water will help the powder dissolve faster.

Pour the formula through a funnel to avoid spillage

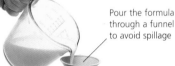

4 Pour the formula milk into the clean bottles through the plastic funnel.

STORING FEEDS

You can make up a batch of feeds that can be stored for 24 hours; this is particularly useful for night feeds. Make up several jugs of formula and pour into bottles. Put the teats on upside down, but don't let them dip into the milk. If they do touch the milk, put the teats the right way up. Cover with the discs and screw on the rings. Cool the bottles and place them in a fridge immediately (but not in the door). Breast milk expressed into bottles can also be stored in this way.

Do not let the teat touch the milk

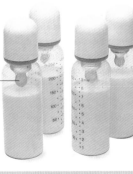

TIME LIMIT
Store prepared formula in the fridge for no longer than 24 hours.

THE FIRST SIX WEEKS

FAMILY CONCERNS

Q HOW DO WE KNOW IF WE WILL MAKE GOOD PARENTS?

A How can any of us know whether we will make good parents? This is something you have to learn "on-the-job", so all you can do is take each day at a time until your confidence grows through experience. Your insecurity may have something to do with the fact that you feel isolated at the moment. Once you have the opportunity to get out more, join a local mother-and-toddler group so that you can share your experiences with others.

Q HOW DO WE COPE WITH EVERYONE GIVING US ADVICE?

A Friends and relatives who have already survived the trials of parenthood, naturally assume that you will want the benefit of their experience. This advice is well-intentioned and often useful but may also be old-fashioned, or conflict with your own ideas of parenthood. It is hard to tell those who mean well that you want to do things your own way, but you must make yourself clear from the outset.

ADJUSTING TO FATHERHOOD

The enormous responsibility of fatherhood, and the fears this evokes, can prevent you from getting the most out of family life initially, but if you learn to play an active role, helping with nappy-changing, bath time, or putting to bed, you will soon feel relaxed and confident with your baby.

Feeling neglected
It's a simple fact that newborn babies can take up every second of a mother's time in the early weeks, and that fathers often feel neglected, or even jealous of the baby. This is only natural because your partner now has a new focus to her life and it is not you. Tell your partner how you feel before this builds up into resentment and causes harm to your relationship. You could also take a more active role in caring for your baby.

Feeling left out
Many new fathers wrongly assume that their partner is coping perfectly well without any help from them but you may be surprised to learn just how much she needs you. Just knowing that you are there helps your partner. If you feel excluded because you cannot share in breastfeeding, perhaps your partner could express some milk into a bottle so that you can help with the feeding too, including in the middle of the night.

Being scared of your baby
Babies seem to be fragile little creatures, and many men are scared to do anything other than hold them unless they have had younger brothers and sisters. Babies are, in fact, quite resilient to inept handling – as long as you don't drop them on their heads. Try to overcome your fears by watching your partner or midwife and then offer to help bathe and change your baby to give your partner a rest.

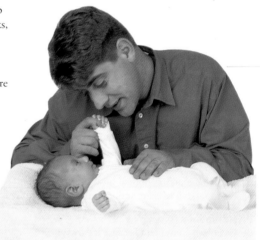

GETTING TO KNOW YOUR BABY
You will come to feel close to your baby through the daily loving contact and care: by changing nappies, giving baths, cuddling, stroking, and talking.

Q HOW WILL OUR OTHER CHILD/ CHILDREN REACT TO THE NEW BABY?

A Other children often see a new arrival as an exciting event. Alternatively, the new arrival may inspire feelings of jealousy in your other offspring; these jealous feelings may not be evident, as you may have expected, straight after the birth, so be prepared to deal with them if they emerge later. There should not be too many problems, as long as your children still get their share of attention and do not feel excluded (see below).

Q HOW CAN WE ENSURE THAT OUR OTHER CHILDREN DO NOT FEEL LEFT OUT?

A As soon as you bring your baby home, try to include your other child or children in everything that's going on by explaining what you are doing, and why, and getting them to help with simple chores. However demanding your new baby is, you should try to make some special time for your other offspring – without the baby – and to honour some of their established routines. For example, if you always read bedtime stories, you or your partner should continue to do so.

Q I FEEL MOODY AND LOW, IS THIS NORMAL?

A In the first few days after the birth you may not feel your usual self; your partner may also be worried that you seem depressed. However, this is quite normal and is probably just a case of the "baby blues" (see p. 218). Physically, you may be tired and sore, and you are possibly mentally overwhelmed by your new responsibility. Your body has undergone an hormonal upheaval, and you may also be anxious about your ability to care for your new baby. Talk to your partner about your feelings, so that he understands how you feel. He too, may be feeling a little exhausted or low as he adjusts to the ups and downs of a newborn baby in his life.

Q I'VE BEEN FEELING DEPRESSED FOR WEEKS, IS THIS NORMAL?

A Although it is normal to feel a bit weepy and low straight after the birth, if these feelings persist beyond the first week, you may be suffering from post-natal depression (see p. 218), which can be a serious problem. You and your partner should talk to your health visitor or doctor about your symptoms, so that you can both understand what you are going through and discuss ways in which you can work together to overcome the depression.

Q HOW CAN MY PARTNER AND I REKINDLE OUR ROMANCE?

A In all the excitement and stress caused by the arrival of your baby, it is easy to neglect each other's needs. It can be difficult to feel romantic in the hectic early round of breastfeeding, changing nappies, and interrupted sleep, but once you have established a routine of caring for your baby, you can begin to think of simple ways to recapture the closeness you and your partner enjoyed before the birth. Ask someone you trust to babysit occasionally so that you and your partner can go out for a meal. Set aside time to express all the mixed feelings you've both had since the arrival of your baby; just cuddle if you are too tired to make love; have a nap or a bath together at the end of the working day; try to make time to give each other a relaxing massage. Be prepared, though, for interruptions!

Q HOW WILL OUR NEW BABY AFFECT OUR SOCIAL LIFE?

A Your baby's demands will naturally take precedence over your social life in these early weeks, although you will probably find that you have plenty of visitors, and that it is also relatively easy to see friends with your new baby. You may also find that you make new friends through your baby as you meet other mothers with young children. Most mothers, however, do not have the energy for late nights at this early stage, but rest assured that your social life will eventually return to a semblance of normality once you all settle into a routine together.

Q WHEN WILL WE SETTLE DOWN AGAIN?

A The first six weeks after the birth are a continual round of bathing, changing, and feeding routines, and you will constantly feel tired. This is the downside of having a newborn baby, but you'll soon begin to experience the joys of parenthood as new patterns become established, as your confidence in handling your baby increases, and as your body begins to make a full recovery from the rigours of pregnancy and labour. You'll also find that your baby will start to distinguish between night (time to sleep) and day (time to wake up and be sociable), which gives you both more time for rest. As your energy returns, your family life will begin to live up to your expectations, and you and your partner will be able to focus on all the positive aspects of parenthood.

CONCERNS ABOUT YOUNG BABIES

Q MY BABY'S FACE IS VERY SPOTTY, IS THIS NORMAL?

A Babies are often spotty but this is rarely serious. Your baby's face may also have small, white spots (milia) caused by hormonal changes. These do not need treatment, and should disappear within a few days or weeks. If the spots are infected and red, leave them alone unless they burst; if this happens, gently clean them with cool, boiled water and apply antiseptic cream. If the infection persists or spreads, consult your doctor.

Q MY BABY'S BOTTOM LOOKS RED AND SORE, WHAT SHOULD I DO?

A Nappy rash is usually caused by the ammonia in urine irritating the skin, so check your baby's nappy often. A young baby's skin is very sensitive, especially to perfumes, chemical products; if a rash (not caused by wet nappies) develops, it may be due to the overuse of, or your baby's sensitivity to products such as baby cream or wipes (especially if they are not hypo-allergenic), and you may have to change or stop using the product. Wash your baby's bottom gently with non-perfumed baby soap and water and pat it dry. Zinc and castor oil cream can ease soreness, and protect against further irritation.

Q MY BABY USUALLY BRINGS UP A LITTLE MILK AFTER A FEED, AM I OVERFEEDING?

A Young babies don't realize when they have had enough milk and often just carry on feeding until they are too full, and then bring up some of their feed. It is also common for babies to vomit when they are trying to get rid of some wind.

Q MY BABY VOMITED WITH GREAT FORCE, IS THIS NORMAL?

A This is called "projectile vomiting". If it happens only once or within 72 hours of the birth, when your baby may still have mucus in his or her stomach, then it is probably not serious. Just feed and wind your baby well (see p. 208). If it happens after every feed, your baby may have a blockage in the outlet of the stomach, known as pyloric stenosis, which needs medical attention. However, this is a very rare condition.

Q WHY IS THERE A BLISTER ON MY BABY'S TOP LIP?

A This is probably a "sucking" blister, caused when the lips tighten around your nipple or a teat. The blister is not serious and needs no treatment; just leave it alone and it should disappear.

HOW DO I PREVENT MY BABY'S FACE GETTING SCRATCHED?

Since babies tend to wave their fists about and touch their faces a lot, they can scratch themselves with the sharp edges of their nails. These scratches are very superficial, and unlikely to cause your baby any lasting harm; they probably cause you more concern because they look sore. To stop this happening, you can buy "scratch" mittens; some stretchsuits have sleeves that cover your baby's hands.

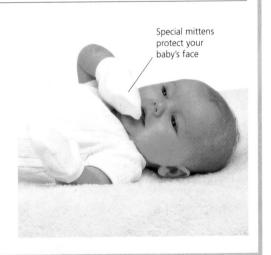

Special mittens protect your baby's face

CUTTING YOUR BABY'S NAILS
Your baby's fingernails are not yet growing independently of the fingers so are not ready to be cut.

Q MY BABY CRIES A LOT AND SEEMS VERY UNCOMFORTABLE, WHAT IS WRONG?

A This may be a condition called colic, which is caused by trapped wind. Colic makes babies cry hard, pull their knees up to their abdomen, and also makes them reluctant to feed or to settle. You can help to relieve the pain by massaging the abdomen, or putting your baby against your shoulder and rubbing the back. Ask your midwife, health visitor, doctor, or a pharmacist at the baby clinic, for medication to ease the colic.

Q MY BABY'S STOOLS ARE VERY LOOSE, IS THIS NORMAL?

A Loose stools are quite common, although babies who are breastfed are much more likely to have looser stools than those who are bottle-fed. However, if your baby's stools are green as well as watery, your baby probably has diarrhoea. This could be serious because it means that your baby is losing fluids, which can lead to dehydration, and this may need medical attention. If your baby has severe diarrhoea, a dry mouth, is lethargic, refuses to feed, and the fontanelle is sunken, contact your doctor at once.

Q WHAT CAN I DO IF MY BABY'S SCALP IS DRY AND SCALY?

A This is a condition called cradle cap, which often occurs in young babies. It looks unpleasant but is not at all serious and shouldn't cause your baby much discomfort. Cradle cap can spread to other parts of your baby's body but usually clears up within a few days. You can treat it by gently rubbing baby oil on to the scalp; leave the oil on for up to 24 hours before using a baby comb to comb the hair and loosen the scales. If, after washing your baby's hair, the scaliness persists, consult your doctor.

Q WHY ARE MY BABY'S EYES STICKY AND "GLUED UP"?

A It is possible that your baby has conjunctivitis, which is a mild eye infection. This can occur in newborn babies if fluid or blood gets into the eye during the delivery. Gently wipe your baby's eyes with cotton wool soaked in cool, boiled water, using a different piece for each eye. If the condition does not clear up, some midwives believe that placing a few drops of breastmilk into the affected eye may help to clear up the infection, but check with your doctor first. If the condition persists, your doctor can prescribe an antibiotic cream.

Q IS OUR SMOKING HARMFUL TO MY YOUNG BABY?

A Yes, a baby's lungs and nose are very sensitive to irritants. Smoke is an irritant, and although your lungs may be used to nicotine, carbon monoxide, and other noxious fumes, your baby's won't be. The fumes from cigarettes paralyse the lining of fine hairs in the nose, throat, and lungs that constantly sweep foreign particles out from the chest and help keep the lungs clear. There may be a link between a very smoky environment and cot death, but smoking around your baby will certainly increase his or her chances of developing respiratory problems such as asthma, chronic cough, and chest infections later on in childhood.

WHEN TO CONSULT A DOCTOR

On occasions your baby is likely to give you cause for concern, but you will soon learn to deal with most situations. However, in any of the situations listed below, your baby will need treatment, and should be taken to a doctor.

Contact your doctor if your baby:
- Is passing green, watery stools.
- Wheezes, and has a dry, rasping cough.
- Has an unusually low temperature.
- Has a skin rash.
- You suspect an infection is present.
- Has been vomiting more than usual.
- Is very lethargic.
- Is generally irritable and is not feeding well.

Contact your doctor or hospital immediately if your baby:
- Is breathing either very quickly, with a noisy grunting sound, or very slowly and irregularly.
- Seems to be having a fit: his or her back is arched and/or the limbs are moving jerkily.
- Has turned blue.
- Is acting strangely and doesn't recognize you, or becomes unrousable or extremely sleepy.
- Has sunken fontanelles.
- Develops a high temperature, especially in conjunction with any of the above.

If you can't contact your doctor, go straight to your local hospital's emergency department or, if you have no transport, ring for an ambulance.

YOUR POST-NATAL CHECK

Q WHY DO I NEED A CHECK-UP AFTER SIX WEEKS?

A Your recovery from pregnancy and labour should be almost complete six weeks after the birth, and your doctor will want to check that everything is returning to normal. By now, your stitches should have healed, your bleeding stopped, and your breasts adapted to feeding, or returned to normal if you are bottle-feeding. If you feel that anything is not quite right, this is an opportunity to get it checked by your doctor.

Q WHEN ARE MY PERIODS LIKELY TO START AGAIN?

A This date varies depending on individual circumstances. Your periods may begin before the post-natal check; if you are bottle-feeding (or you breastfeed only for a short time), your periods should return between two and four months after the birth but if you breastfeed for longer, your periods may not return until your baby starts to take solid food, or possibly even later.

Q WHEN DO I NEED TO START THINKING ABOUT CONTRACEPTION?

A Straight away, because even though your periods haven't started yet, it is important to realize that you could become pregnant again within a month or two of giving birth because ovulation can occur before your first period. Although breastfeeding reduces the likelihood of this, it is not a reliable form of contraception.

Q WHAT METHODS OF CONTRACEPTION CAN I USE?

A Condoms, diaphragms, and all barrier methods of contraception are safe to use at any time. You can take the Pill if you are bottle-feeding, but if you have chosen to breastfeed, your doctor will advise against hormonal contraception as oestrogen can inhibit milk production. The "Mini-pill" (containing only progesterone) is compatible with breastfeeding, but must be taken at the same time every day to be effective. There is also an electronic monitor available; this tests your urine for hormones, and shows the days when you are ovulating and those when you are safe. However, this system should not be used if you are breastfeeding.

WHAT HAPPENS AT THE POST-NATAL CHECK?

As well as a physical examination to check that you are fully recovered, the post-natal check is an ideal time to discuss any problems or incidents that occurred during your pregnancy or labour and why these occurred, and to express any other worries you may have (see opposite). It is normally carried out either at your doctor's surgery or at the hospital clinic; however, if you had a Caesarean, high blood pressure (pre-eclampsia), or any other complications, you will usually have to see the consultant at your hospital. Your doctor will also discuss your choice of birth control method.

Checks and advice
Any or all of the following checks will be carried out and appropriate advice given:
■ Your urine is tested for protein, to check your kidney function and for urinary tract infection.
■ Your weight is recorded.
■ Your blood pressure noted.
■ Your breasts and nipples are checked, especially if your are breastfeeding.
■ Your abdomen is examined to check that your womb has shrunk back to its normal size.
■ Any wounds (Caesarean or episiotomy) are examined.
■ Your vagina and perineum are examined.
■ You may be offered a cervical smear test if you have not had one recently, or if the last one gave an abnormal result.
■ If there is any suspicion that you are anaemic, blood will be taken to test haemoglobin levels.
■ If you are not immune to rubella (German measles), you will be offered a vaccination.
■ You will be given advice about contraception: depending on your preference, you can have a new coil inserted or a new cap fitted; you can go on the "Mini-pill" (see left) or be given condoms.

I'M WORRIED ABOUT...

This is an excellent time to discuss with your doctor any health issues that you are concerned about, or any embarrassing problems that you are experiencing – from soreness to your sex life. It will also put your mind at rest to discover that your fears and problems are very common and also easily remedied.

I am still sore in the perineal area

If you had an episiotomy (cut) or tear in the perineal area at the birth, the stitches should have dissolved, and the wound should have healed by now. If the area is still red or feels sore, there may be an infection present, and your doctor (or possibly an obstetrician) will check this now; you may need to take an antibiotic to help clear up the infection. Sometimes, if the stitches haven't dissolved properly, they have to be removed by the doctor.

My vagina feels different

It is common to feel that your vaginal area is "different" after having a baby and to some extent this is true: your pelvic floor muscles have been stretched and need to be exercised to regain their original elasticity (see p. 222). Some women fear that they have not been stitched back together properly. Although this is most unlikely, in extremely rare cases where the stitches have healed badly, the result can interfere with the ability to pass water and hold wind properly and even mar your sex life. In this case it may be necessary to have an operation, called a "refashioning of the perineum", to return things to normal.

I am leaking urine

Many women experience urine leakage (stress incontinence) after childbirth, so don't be embarrassed to talk about it. Most commonly it settles within a few weeks. The sooner you bring it to your doctor's attention the sooner you will be referred to a specialist unit if this is necessary. Usually it is the result of damaged or weak pelvic floor muscles.

Sometimes exercises can help, or a simple treatment is all that is required. Infection can also make you leak, so a urine specimen is often asked for, or a course of antibiotics prescribed.

I feel weak after my Caesarean

If you had a Caesarean delivery, your stomach muscles can take some time to knit back together again and you will not have much strength in your abdominal area. You should avoid any lifting or driving for the first six weeks to give the wound time to heal properly; it will be at least three months before you can lift heavy objects, run, or take up sport again. Apart from the pelvic tilt (see p. 222), avoid any exercise until after six weeks.

I feel so tired

Many women feel exhausted in the weeks after the birth because of broken nights, but if your fatigue is accompanied by breathlessness and pallor, you may be anaemic. This can be caused by a lack of iron, or a loss of blood during labour. Normal blood loss does not cause a problem because your body rapidly makes up the oxygen-carrying blood cells. If you had a Caesarean, you may have lost twice as much blood as after a vaginal delivery, so you may need to take iron tablets to replenish your body's stores.

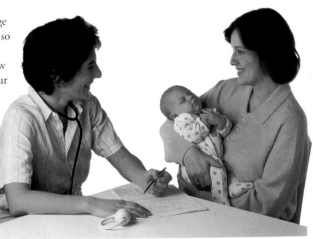

A SYMPATHETIC EAR
Your doctor will be ready to discuss any problems you are experiencing during your recovery.

THE FIRST SIX WEEKS

YOUR BABY'S SIX-WEEK CHECK

Q HOW HAS MY BABY DEVELOPED OVER THE FIRST SIX WEEKS?

A You will find that your baby has become a more responsive individual, and less of a noisy, demanding bundle. You may also find that he or she does not cry as much as before, and that there is a longer wakeful period during the day. Control over the limbs has increased and the fists have unclenched, enabling objects to be grasped more easily. You will notice how your baby enjoys kicking his or her legs in the air. When lying face down, your baby may be able to lift his or her head momentarily, but will remain unable to do this when sitting.

WHICH IMMUNIZATIONS AND CHECKS WILL MY BABY NEED?

The six-week check is the first part of your baby's medical programme and is followed by check-ups and vaccinations up to four years old. Some vaccines are long-lasting, others need to be boosted at regular intervals. Call the Department of Health for a schedule (see p. 232).

Immunizations

AGE	IMMUNIZATION
2, 3, 4 months	DTP – Diphtheria, tetanus, polio, pertussis (whooping cough)
12 – 15 months	MMR – Measles, mumps, rubella
3 – 4 years	Pre-school booster of MMR, plus polio, diphtheria, and tetanus

Check-ups

■ At eight months, your baby's hearing, growth, and development are tested.
■ At two years, your baby's walking, talking, comprehension, and co-ordination (fine motor skills) are assessed.
■ At three-and-a-half years, the physical development, speech, and hearing are checked.

Q CAN MY BABY RECOGNIZE ME OR MY PARTNER YET?

A Yes, one of the biggest thrills for you and your partner is that your baby now has a range of facial expressions and can respond to you both. Your baby's head turns upon hearing your voice, and he or she will stare at your face when you are talking, meeting your eyes and smiling at you.

Q IS IT NORMAL FOR A PREMATURE BABY TO BE REALLY DIFFICULT AT FIRST?

A Premature babies can be especially difficult during the first six weeks, crying incessantly and refusing to be comforted, no matter how hard you try, or be very sleepy and reluctant to feed. He or she needs extra care, more frequent feeding, and lots of warmth – but because there is less response you may feel rejected. As he or she matures, you will see a reaction to your care. The check-up is a good time to ask about any problems that are causing you anxiety.

Q CAN IMMUNIZATIONS REALLY CAUSE BRAIN DAMAGE?

A There have been alarming stories about the side-effects of vaccinations, but these cases are rare. There is no firm evidence that immunizations cause brain inflammation (encephalitis) and brain damage. Some babies and children have developed fits and subsequent brain damage shortly after being immunized, but as these problems afflict some babies anyway – even if they are not immunized – it may well be a matter of chance that some of them had received immunizations only a few days earlier.

QUESTIONS TO ASK

Is my baby developing normally?

Can my baby see and hear properly?

How do I get information about immunization?

Can I delay the start of the vaccination programme?

Do I have to remember check-up dates or will I be reminded?

WHAT IS THE DOCTOR LOOKING FOR?

The six-week check is the first of the major developmental assessments for a new baby. Your doctor or local baby clinic will carry out the check in relaxed surroundings. This is a good time to raise any queries you may have about the daily care of your baby.

ROUTINE CHECKS

Your baby is undressed so that the doctor can observe how he or she moves her limbs. Your baby will be examined in detail from head to foot to ensure that physical progress is normal, and you will be asked questions about your baby's feeding and toilet habits, as well as general well-being.

General assessment
The head circumference is measured to check for normal growth, and the fontanelles (soft parts of your baby's head at the front and back where the skull bones meet) are checked for abnormalities. His or her eyes, ears, and mouth are examined; the chest and breathing are checked, and the genitals inspected. The doctor will also feel your baby's abdomen to ensure that the liver, stomach, and spleen are all developing normally; by manipulating your baby's legs, the hips are checked for possible dislocation.

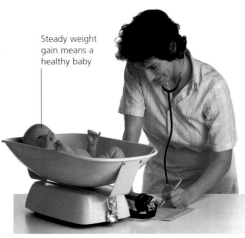

Steady weight gain means a healthy baby

WEIGHING
Your baby will be weighed regularly and the weight gain compared with the birth weight. Normal weight gain usually means a healthy baby; the weight chart will be an important record for months to come.

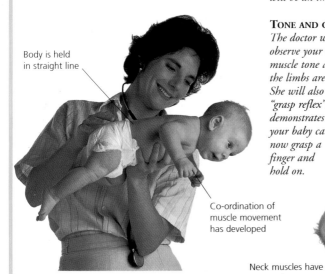

Body is held in straight line

Co-ordination of muscle movement has developed

CONTROL OF HEAD
Now that your baby has some control over the neck muscles, the doctor will see if he or she holds the head in line with the body while being held in the air, and even when moved into a sitting position.

TONE AND GRASP
The doctor will observe your baby's muscle tone and how the limbs are working. She will also check the "grasp reflex", which demonstrates that your baby can now grasp a finger and hold on.

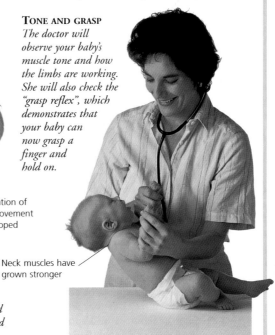

Neck muscles have grown stronger

THE FIRST SIX WEEKS

YOUR RIGHTS AND BENEFITS

As soon as you become pregnant you are eligible for certain rights and benefits (see below). To claim these, you should get the appropriate forms from your midwife, doctor's surgery, or local Social Security office. There are deadlines by which you should apply for your benefits, so check the Rights and Benefits Summary (see below, opposite) to ensure that you do not miss out. Soon after the birth, you must register your baby's name and birth at a register office (see opposite). Your rights concerning maternity leave are outlined below.

BENEFITS

■ You are entitled to free NHS dental care and free prescriptions while pregnant and for a year after your baby is born.
■ If you are on a low income, check with the your local Social Security office whether you are entitled to free eye tests, vouchers towards your spectacles, assistance with travel to your hospital, as well as free milk and vitamins.

■ If you or your partner are on Income Support, are unemployed, or are disabled, you may be entitled to a single payment of £100 to help buy necessities for your baby (called a Maternity Payment).
■ Child benefit is a tax-free weekly benefit given irrespective of National Insurance contributions or income. You must register for it within six months of your baby's birth; it will be backdated to the birth date.

IF YOU WORK

If you work for an employer, talk to your employer as soon as possible about your maternity leave and pay. At least 21 days before you intend to stop work, you should confirm in writing to your employer the date you intend to leave, when your baby is due, and when you are planning to return to work. This will protect your right to Statutory Maternity Pay (SMP). If you are self-employed, you are not entitled to SMP, but you may be entitled to a Maternity Allowance. These are both payable for up to 18 weeks.

Maternity leave
■ You are entitled by law to at least 14 weeks' maternity leave, as long as you notify your employer in writing at least 21 days before your maternity leave starts, and your job must be kept open for your return.
■ The earliest date that maternity leave can start is 11 weeks before the week your baby is due.
■ If, by the eleventh week before the expected week of confinement, you have worked for your employer for two years, you can remain on maternity leave until 28 weeks after the birth.
■ During your pregnancy, while you are still at work, you are entitled to take paid time off to attend your antenatal clinics and classes.
■ When you are pregnant you are also protected under the Employment Protection Act against unfair dismissal for maternity-related reasons. If you are suspended from your job for health or safety reasons,

your employer is legally obliged to offer you another suitable position or to give you full pay during the period of suspension.
■ To protect your right to return to work, you should write to your employer three weeks before you intend to return to confirm the date.
■ By law, if you have still not returned to work 29 weeks after the birth of your baby, you may lose your right to return to your previous job.

Statutory Maternity Pay
You are entitled to SMP if you have been working for the same company for 26 weeks by the fifteenth week before the week your baby is due, and have earned enough to pay class 1 National Insurance. You will receive 90 per cent of your average weekly earnings for the first six weeks and a flat rate for the next 12 weeks.

Maternity Allowance
If you can't get Statutory Maternity Pay because perhaps you have recently given up your job, or changed jobs, or you are self-employed, you may be able to claim up to 18 weeks' Maternity Allowance. Check with the Social Security office for the qualifying rules. You will normally be paid for a core period of 13 weeks beginning six weeks before the week your baby is due. If you are unemployed or sick, check with your Social Security office whether you qualify for a Maternity Allowance.

REGISTERING YOUR BABY'S BIRTH

You must register your baby's birth with the Registrar of Births, Deaths, and Marriages within six weeks in England, Northern Ireland, and Wales, and within three weeks in Scotland. Go to the register office local to the hospital where your baby was born because the hospital will have sent details of your baby there. You will be given a birth certificate and a form that will enable you to get a medical card with a National Health Service number so that you can register your baby with your doctor, and a child benefit claim form.

What you need to know

If you are married, only one of you needs to see the registrar. If you are not married to the baby's father and you want his details on the birth certificate, the father must be with you. You must be absolutely clear about your baby's name; if you wish to change even minor details, like the spelling, after the certificate has been issued, you will have to pay for a new certificate, and you can do this only once. A basic certificate is free but there is a more elaborate version for a small fee.

A father's rights

If you are married to the mother of your child, you will have a right to be registered as the father on your child's birth certificate. If you are not married to the mother but you wish to be registered as the father, you must both attend at the registering of the birth

Registering a stillbirth or a baby who has died

If your baby was stillborn after 24 weeks or died after the birth (regardless of how premature he or she was) your baby should still be registered so that you can get a certificate of burial. You are also still entitled to all benefits, including free prescriptions, dental treatment, Maternity Allowance, and SMP if your baby dies.

RIGHTS AND BENEFITS SUMMARY

WHEN	WHAT TO DO	WHY
As soon as you know you are pregnant	▪ If you are working, inform your employer ▪ Find out if you are entitled to Maternity Allowance (MA)	▪ To establish eligibility for SMP; for paid time off for antenatal visits ▪ If you are not eligible for SMP
3 weeks before intending to stop work	▪ Confirm to your employer in writing when you will stop work, also your return date	▪ To protect your right to return to work; and to get SMP
14 weeks before the week your baby is due	▪ Ask your doctor/midwife for a maternity certificate (MAT B1)	▪ Your employer needs this
11 weeks before the week your baby is due	▪ You can leave work from this date	▪ SMP and Maternity Allowance are paid if you have stopped work
As soon after the birth as possible	▪ Register the baby's birth ▪ Apply for Child Benefit	▪ To get a birth certificate, form for an NHS card, and child benefit form
By 6 weeks after the birth (3 weeks in Scotland)	▪ You should have registered the baby's birth	▪ This is the latest date
7 weeks after the baby was due	▪ Write to your employer to confirm that you are returning to work	▪ To protect your right to return to work
3 weeks before returning to work	▪ Write to your employer with date of return to work	▪ To protect your right to return to work
6 months after the birth	▪ The latest date to claim Child Benefit and get it backdated to the birth	▪ You cannot backdate this more than 6 months
29 weeks after the birth	▪ The latest date to return to work	▪ You may lose your right to return

GLOSSARY

Abruption Premature separation of the placenta from the wall of the womb.

Amniocentesis A procedure in which a small sample of amniotic fluid is removed from around the baby.

Amniotic fluid The fluid surrounding your baby (known as the waters).

Amniotomy (artificial rupture of membranes ARM) Breaking the membranes using a special plastic hook.

Anaemia Lack of haemoglobin in red blood cells, due to iron deficiency or disease.

Antenatal Before birth.

Antepartum haemorrhage (APH) Vaginal bleeding that happens after 24 weeks of pregnancy and before delivery.

Anti-D An injection of antibodies given to women whose blood group is Rhesus negative, if there is a chance that they have been exposed to fetal blood cells.

Breech The baby is lying bottom down in the womb.

Cardiotocograph (CTG) An electronic monitor used to record the baby's heartbeat and the mother's contractions.

Cephalic The baby is lying head down in the womb.

Chorion villus sampling (CVS) A method for sampling placental tissue for genetic or chromosome studies.

Cilia The fine hairs that line the Fallopian tubes.

Cordocentesis The procedure for taking blood from the baby's umbilical cord via a needle through the abdomen.

Cystitis Infection of the bladder.

Dizygous Non-identical (fraternal) twins.

Doppler A form of ultrasound used specifically to investigate blood flow in the placenta or in the baby.

Down's syndrome (trisomy 21) A disorder caused by the presence of an extra chromosome (21) in the cells.

Ectopic pregnancy A pregnancy that develops outside of the womb.

Embryo The medical term for the baby from conception to about six weeks.

Epidural anaesthesia A method of numbing the nerves of the lower spinal cord to ensure a pain-free labour.

Episiotomy A cut of the perineum and vagina performed by a midwife or doctor to make the delivery easier.

Fallopian tubes Two tubular structures (one on each side of the womb) leading from the ovaries to the womb.

Fetus Medical term for the baby from six weeks after conception until birth.

Fibroid A benign (non-cancerous) growth of muscle of the womb, usually spherically shaped.

Forceps Metal instruments that fit on either side of the baby's head and are used to help deliver the baby.

Fundus The top of the womb.

Haemoglobin (Hb) The oxygen-carrying constituent of red blood cells.

Hepatitis Viruses (named A, B, C, E, and others) that infect the liver, causing jaundice and generalized illness.

Hypertension High blood pressure.

Induction of labour (IOL) The procedure for starting off labour artificially.

In utero death (IUD) The death of the unborn baby after 24 weeks.

In vitro fertilization (IVF) A method of assisted conception in which fertilization occurs in a "test tube" and the embryo is replaced in the womb.

Lanugo The fine hair that covers the fetus in the womb.

Liquor See amniotic fluid.

Lochia Blood loss after the birth.

Membranes Two sets of protective sacs enclosing the baby, called the amnion and the chorion.

Miscarriage The loss of a baby before 24 weeks of pregnancy.

Monozygous Identical twins.

Neonatal A baby less than 28 days old.

Nuchal scan A special ultrasound scan that can check for Down's syndrome.

Oedema Swelling of the fingers, legs, toes, and face.

Oocyte One egg that is released from the ovary at each ovulation.

Placenta A flat, thick disc-shaped organ that supplies the fetus with oxygen and nutrients.

Placenta praevia A placenta situated over, or near to, the cervix which makes a vaginal delivery unlikely.

Post-natal After birth.

Postpartum haemorrhage (PPH) Excessive bleeding following delivery.

Pre-eclampsia A condition that features high blood pressure, oedema, and proteinuria. May be mild or serious.

Presentation Describes the way the baby is lying in the womb.

Preterm (premature) labour Labour before 37 weeks of pregnancy.

Puerperium Just after and up to six weeks after delivery.

Rhesus(Rh) factor Blood is either Rhesus positive or Rhesus negative.

Spinal anaesthesia An injection of anaesthetic into the spine for pain relief in labour (similar to an epidural).

Stillbirth Birth of a baby after 24 weeks of pregnancy who shows no signs of life.

Sutures Stitches.

Thrombosis A blood clot, commonly occurring in the calf; most dangerous if in the lungs (pulmonary embolus).

Toxoplasmosis A parasite infection that can be caught from cats or other pets.

Transverse The baby is lying sideways in the womb.

Urinary tract infection (UTI) Infection affecting the kidneys and/or bladder.

Uterus Womb.

Vernix Thick, greasy substance covering the baby's skin in the womb.

INDEX

Page numbers in italic refer to illustrations

MEDICAL REFERENCES

The papers listed below will give you an opportunity to read for yourself the original papers that help to shape obstetric practice.

Ultrasound scanning: safety and usefulness
Crane J P, LeFevre M L, Winborn R C, et al. A randomized trial of prenatal ultrasonographic screening: impact on the detection, management and outcome of anomalous fetuses. The RADIUS Study Group. *American Journal of Obstetrics and Gynecology* 1994; vol. 172: pp. 382–9
Grisso J A, Strom B L, Cosmatos I, et al. Diagnostic ultrasound in pregnancy and low birthweight. *American Journal of Perinatology* 1994; vol. 11: pp. 297–301
Newnham J P, Evans Michael, C A, et al. Effects of frequent ultrasound during pregnancy: a randomized controlled trial. *The Lancet* 1993; vol. 342: pp. 878–91

Screening for Down's syndrome
Nicolaides K H, Brizot M L, Snijders R J M. Fetal nuchal translucency thickness: ultrasound screening for fetal trisomy in the first trimester of pregnancy. *British Journal of Obstetrics and Gynaecology* 1994; vol. 101: pp. 782–786
Wald N J, Cuckle H S, Densem J W et al. Maternal serum screening for Down's Syndrome in early pregnancy. *British Medical Journal* 1988; vol. 297: pp. 883–887

Methods for reducing the risk of postpartum haemorrhage
Irons D W, Sriskandalaban P, Bullough C H. A simple alternative to parenteral oxytocics for the third stage of labour. *International Journal of Gynaecology and Obstetrics* 1994; vol. 46: pp. 15–18
McDonald S J, Prendiville W J, Blair E. Randomized controlled trial of oxytocin alone versus oxytocin and ergometrine in active management of the third stage of labour. *British Medical Journal* 1993; vol. 307: pp. 1167–71

Yuen P M, Chan N S, Yim S F, et al. A randomized double blind comparison of syntometrine and syntocinon in the management of the third stage of labour. *British Journal of Obstetrics and Gynaecology* 1995; vol. 102: pp. 377–80

Vitamin K and the baby: safety and reasons for use
Grant, J M. Treating all babies with vitamin K: an "unnatural" policy? (editorial). *British Journal of Obstetrics and Gynaecology* 1996; vol. 103: p. xxii
von Kries R, Gobel U, Hachmeister A, et al. Vitamin K and childhood cancer: a population based case-control study in lower Saxony, Germany. *British Medical Journal* 1996; vol. 313: pp. 199–203

Forceps and ventouse usage
Hillier C E, Johanson R B. Worldwide survey of assisted vaginal delivery. *International Journal of Gynaecology and Obstetrics* 1994; vol. 47: pp. 109–14
Sultan A H, Kamm M A, Hudson C N, Bartram C I. Anal sphincter disruption during vaginal delivery. *New England Journal of Medecine* 1993; vol. 329: pp. 1905–1911

Electronic fetal heart rate monitoring in labour
Grant A, O'Brian N, Joy M T, et al. Cerebral palsy among children born during the Dublin randomized trial of intrapartum fetal monitoring. *The Lancet* 1989; vol. ii: pp. 1233–36
Mahomed K, Nyoni R, Malumbo T et al. Randomized controlled trial of intrapartum fetal heart rate monitoring. *British Medical Journal* 1994; vol. 308: pp. 497–500

Vaginal delivery after previous Caesarean section
Flamm B J, Janice R G, Liu Y, Wolde Tzadik G. Elective repeat Caesarean delivery versus trial of labour: a prospective multicentre study. *Obstetrics and Gynecology* 1994; vol. 83: pp. 927–932

ACKNOWLEDGMENTS

The authors would like to thank:

Christoph Lees would like to thank Deb and Patrick Conner, Hugh and Patricia Sergeant for their helpful comments and input; to Trish Chudleigh; Dr Edward Petch for advice on mental illness in pregnancy; Dr Lesley Roberts for scouring the text and posing for photographs. Finally, thanks to the staff in the obstetric units at Greenwich and King's Hospitals who, although they may not realize it, inspired this book. Grainne McCartan would like to thank her parents Marion and Xavier; also Gretta Duffy, Xavier McCartan, Sen, Brian, Kim, Patsy, Jenny, Juliet, Peter, Sandra, Linda, Briege, Shirley, Alicia, and Jack for all their help and support.

Dorling Kindersley would like to thank the following:

DESIGN ASSISTANCE Jennifer Bayliss, Sue Callister, Evan Jones, Claudine Meissner, Kylie Mulquin.

EDITORIAL ASSISTANCE Fergus Collins, Maureen Rissik, Katherine Robinson, Debbie Voller, Pippa Ward.

DTP ASSISTANCE Ian Merrill, Rachel Symons.

ILLUSTRATORS Joanna Cameron, Karen Cochrane, Sandie Hill, Paul Richardson, Gill Tomblin, Halli Verrinder.

PICTURE CREDITS Collections/Anthea Sieveking 149 br, 168cl, c, cr, 169l, r, 174br, 188br; Sally Greenhill: 37 l, 158 bl; Oxford

Scientific Film: /Derek Bromhall 57tr; Science Photo Library: /BSIP VEM 51tr; /Dr. Jeremy Burgess 61tr; /J. Croyle/Custom Medical Stock 88; /Joseph Nettis 215br; /Petit Format/Nestle 8tl, 42, 49tr, 59tr; /Row Sutherland 183br.
Every effort has been made to trace the copyright holders and we apologize in advance for any unintentional omissions. We would be pleased to insert the appropriate acknowledgment in any subsequent edition of this publication.

ADDITIONAL PHOTOGRAPHY Eddie Lawrence.

MODELS Sue Berry, Amber Bezer, Ellie Blancke, Tracey Blancke, Emma Burt, Angie Callan, Sue Callister, Louise Clairmont, Roberto Costa, Felicity Crowe, Duane Duncan, Jo Evans, Yvette Fernandez, Lee Goodger, Joany Haig, Toby Judge, Leesa Kotting, Silvia Lagreca, Andrew Lecoyte, Shahida Majeed, Ian Merrill, Mutsumi Niwa, Kelly Priestly, Eleanor Roberts, Leslie Roberts, Katherine Robinson, Charlie Rutherford, Derek Rutherford, Ellena Rutherford, Faye Rutherford, Jo-anne Skinner, Shannon Skinner, Emily Wood.

MAKE-UP Karen Fundell, Lynn Percival.

HOME ECONOMIST Alison Austin.

PROPS John Bell & Croydon, Kings Health Care NHS Trust.

CLOTHES AND EQUIPMENT supplied with thanks to Mothercare, Blooming Marvellous, Bumpsadaisy, Early Learning Centre.